"Mina Dobic is an intuitive woman comr
humanity and One Peaceful World. Growing
motivated by a sincere desire to fulfil her goal, sh
transform their sicknesses and misery into health, happiness and peace.:

Mr. Michio Kushi, acknowledged leader of the
International Macrobiotic Community and Natural Foods Movement

"Mina's story of her life is moving as well as amazing. Her journey from Yugoslavia to Becket, Massachusetts, to California and how she overcame her own cancer, has inspired others who are sick to seek her help. Her healing advice has seen me through many of my illnesses with her love, compassion and insights. This book will make it possible for many more to hear her story and learn her wisdom of healing."

Dr. Benjamin Spock, Pediatrician and Author

"I am overwhelmed by the beauty, insight, and courage of this book. Mina is a special kind of healer. This book will give you a wonderful tool for maintaining your health. It will also give you a refreshing and insightful way of looking at any health challenge.'

Bill Duke, Hollywood Director, Actor, Author

"Mina Dobic, a macrobiotic expert who advised Hollywood celebrities and teaches classes throughout Southern California…"

The San Diego Union Tribune, April 29, 1998

"Mina Dobic is widely considered L.A.'s most expert macrobiotic health consultant."

Vogue Magazine, May 1997

"Considered one of the leading experts in the field of macrobiotics, Mina Dobic's *Wellness through Macrobiotics* cooking seminars at The Ritz-Carlton, Laguna Niguel, have been a tremendous source of help to hundreds of individuals. The informational cooking classes, lectures and lunches emphasize the healing power of food, how food can increase energy and strengthen health. Working alongside and training chefs in the techniques of macrobiotic cooking, Mina stresses the importance of designing daily menus to balance changing seasons. Mina truly is in the business of saving lives through changes in lifestyles and healthy eating. The results are dramatic and indisputable.

Ashley Goodwin, Manager of Special Events,
the Ritz-Carlton, Laguna Niguel

"With boundless love and wisdom, Mina guided me on my macrobiotic journey to recovery from metastatic breast cancer. Now through her book, many others' lives will be touched by this powerhouse of a woman whose kitchen is her primary resource for healing. Her story is a message of hope for everyone facing life-threatening illness, particularly those on whom the medical community has given up."

Jennifer E. Greene, Ph.D.

My Beautiful Life

My Beautiful Life

"HOW MACROBIOTICS
BROUGHT ME FROM CANCER
TO RADIANT HEALTH."

Milenka 'Mina' Dobic

FINDHORN
Press

First published in 2000

ISBN 1 899171 13 4

British Library Cataloguing-in-Publication Data.
A catalogue record for this book is available from the British Library.

Library of Congress Catalog Card Number: 99-67783

Layout by Pam Bochel
Front cover design by Dale Vermeer

Printed and bound in the USA

Published by
Findhorn Press

The Park, Findhorn   P.O. Box 13939
Forres IV36 3TY   Tallahassee
Scotland   Florida 32317-3939, USA
Tel 01309 690582   Tel 850 893 2920
Fax 01309 690036   Fax 850 893 3442
e-mail info@findhornpress.com
findhornpress.com

Dedication

With the deepest veneration to the memory of Katarina and Kaja Popov, my mother and father, who inspired me and taught me the love of peace.

With the utmost gratefulness to my dear friend Ratka Rudic, M.D. for guiding me to the light when I was immersed in my own darkness.

With unconditional love to my guardian angels, who support me and all who need it, my husband Bosko, my son Srdjan and my daughter Yelena.

With honor to Michio and Aveline Kushi, my dear teachers, whose lives are the very cornerstone for the creation of a more healthy and peaceful world. Thank you for the discernment, insight and knowledge which led me and my family to find the way to that healthy and peaceful world.

Disclaimer

To the Reader:

Those with health problems are advised to seek the guidance of a qualified medical or psychological professional in addition to a qualified macrobiotic counselor before implementing any of the dietary and other approaches presented in this book. It is essential that any readers who have any reason to suspect serious illness in themselves or their family members seek appropriate medical, nutritional, or psychological advice promptly. Neither this or any other health related book should be used as a substitute for qualified care or treatment.

This book is sold with the understanding that the author and publisher are not liable for the misconception or misuse of the information provided. The author and publisher shall have neither liability nor responsibility to any person or entity with respect to any loss, damage, or injury caused or alleged to be caused directly or indirectly by the information contained in this book.

Table of Contents

Foreword   11

Preface   15

Introduction   17

Chapter 1   "The Year of Hope: The Year of Salvation"
             Roots of a Cherished Life   21

Chapter 2   Loving What I Do   33

Chapter 3   Private Bliss and Disappointment   39

Chapter 4   My Cancer is a Blessing   49

Chapter 5   Choosing the Macrobiotic Way   59

Chapter 6   Home from the Hospital   67

Chapter 7   First Trip to U.S.: A Celebration of Life!   73

Chapter 8   Michio Kushi   87

Chapter 9   Macrobiotics in Yugoslavia: The Phoenix Rises   93

Chapter 10   Becket: Training for Future Career   109

Chapter 11   California Dream   127

Chapter 12   Healing Stories   135

Appendix A   Back to Basics   165

Appendix B   Menu Used by Mina Dobic to Heal Her Cancer   175

Glossary   184

Bibliography   187

Directories   189

Acknowledgments   190

Foreword

We are facing a grave biological and psychological crisis in human society on this planet, because the modern lifestyle of our current civilization has developed unnaturally, causing changes in dietary patterns.

In the twentieth century, especially during its latter period, the progress of artificialization, chemicalization and industrialization of food have advanced throughout the world. Together with environmental contamination, this trend towards dietary change has been creating heart disease, cancer, arthritis, allergies, diabetes, and various types of viral diseases, as well as psychological and emotional instability among modern people.

In order to restore the proper human diet and realize planetary health and peace, macrobiotic understanding based upon traditional, universal common sense has offered a solution for this crisis of mankind. Since the 1960s, it has innovated the natural, organic food movement and it has initiated alternative medicine of various kinds.

Macrobiotic education began among the grass roots and it has penetrated gradually but steadily among all levels of society during its forty years. In addition it has also spread to every major country during this period. Hundreds of thousands of people have received physical and psychological benefits including recovery from many disorders. One of the remarkable stories of such a recovery is the story of Mina Dobic.

Mina and her husband Bosko, together with their lovely, strong children, are contributing to One Peaceful World, which is a goal of macrobiotics. One Peaceful World is not a visibly-structured social system but it is a brotherhood and sisterhood of every individual on this planet as a family member in health, love, and peace.

Mina and her family are one of the centers from which the light of One Peaceful World radiates out over many thousands of people, through their presence, talking, meeting, cooking classes, writing, and the gathering of their friends.

Michio Kushi
Brookline, Massachusetts
February 10, 1998

In recognition of the role macrobiotics has played in stimulating the natural foods movement and the health revolution in American society, The National Museum of American History, Smithsonian Institute has approved the acquisition of our life's work, establishing an archive of macrobiotic papers and associated materials. These materials will be made available to researchers, students and the general public free of charge, as part of the national collection. This autumn, Mina and Bosko Dobic organized the first in a nationwide series of fund-raising dinners to establish the Kushi Collection at the Smithsonian Institution in Washington, DC.

I remember the Laguna Niguel party vividly. Local macrobiotic chefs and the Executive Chef of The Ritz Carlton Hotel in Dana Point devoted many hours preparing a magnificent banquet. Chris Akbar and Patricio Garcia de Paredes, two young macrobiotic teachers, accompanied Michio and me.

About a hundred people, including well know personalities, enjoyed the buffet, entertainment and conversation. One woman sang a Russian folk song that I used to sing in college and it brought back fond memories.

I was delighted to see how young and beautiful Mina looked. I had not seen her for nearly a decade. She spoke eloquently and clearly, everyone admired her. My mind went back nearly eleven years ago when I first met Mina in Yugoslavia. She had been diagnosed with fourth-stage ovarian cancer and presented a very sad, dark countenance. Following her diagnosis, Mina decided to forgo Western medicine's techniques of radiation and chemotherapy and seek healing through a macrobiotic lifestyle. Following our seminars there, she and her family eventually moved to America and studied with us at the Kushi Institute.

As Michio always says, family support is the most important factor in getting well. Mina's husband, Bosko, helped her so much. He is very strong and, together with their two children, worked tirelessly at the Kushi Institute in Becket, Massachusetts. They assisted with cooking, cleaning, driving and other arrangements, soon making themselves indispensable. Mina soon became one of our head chefs, cooking for cancer patients. As a result of their influence, hundreds of their countrymen came to study in Becket, and the Dobics welcomed and translated for them during their visits.

After completing their studies at the Kushi Institute, they moved to California. Mina has become an outstanding teacher, counselor, and chef who inspires and guides many people to greater health and happiness. As her book reveals, she is a shining example of the macrobiotic spirit and an international treasure for the health of the world.

The success of macrobiotics is due, in no small part, to the Dobics and many wonderful people from many countries and cultures. Without them, knowledge of the healing qualities of a macrobiotic diet would not have spread so rapidly.

Aveline Kushi
Brookline, Massachusetts
December 20, 1997

Michio Kushi is the founder and president of the East West Foundation, a non-profit, educational and cultural institution and recognized leader of the natural foods movement. He has written several books including *The Macrobiotic Approach to Cancer, Macrobiotics and Oriental Medicine,* and *How to See Your Health: Book of Oriental Diagnosis and One Peaceful World.*

Aveline is the wife of Michio Kushi and mother of 5 children. She is a superb macrobiotic cook and teacher, and author of many books on macrobiotics including *Complete Guide to Macrobiotic Cooking, Macrobiotic Diet* and *Aveline: The Life and Dream of the Woman Behind Macrobiotics Today.*

Preface

The story of Mina Dobic and her family is a modern American odyssey. Her journey to health and wholeness weaves together many of the transcendent themes of the last half century; the struggle between communism and a free society, the conflict between conventional medicine and holistic health and the centrifugal forces pulling apart the modern family and the unifying thread that serves to hold it all together.

Along the way Mina passed from cancer victim to cancer survivor, from patient to healer, from student to teacher. Today she is one of the leading macrobiotic cooks and counsellors on the West Coast, inspiring many others with her wisdom, love and compassion.

Thanks to the Dobics and many other families around the world macrobiotics is beginning to enter the mainstream and influence the course of modern society. Recent developments include:

- The National Institute of Health (NIH), the U.S. government's highest medical research organization is presently researching the macrobiotic approach to cancer through a grant awarded to the University of Minnesota in cooperation with the Kushi Institute

- The U.S. Department of Agriculture issued national standards for organic food for the first time, officially recognizing the superiority of chemically-free foods introduced by the Kushis and their associates over thirty years ago

- The Smithsonian Institution in Washington, D.C. is planning to open the Kushi Collection, an exhibit of macrobiotic books, foods and cookware, in recognition of the role of macrobiotics in the current health and diet revolution

- The Ritz-Carlton Hotels, the Prince Hotels and other international chains are serving macrobiotic food in their dining rooms around the world

- The Kellogg School of Management at Northwestern University in Evanston, Ill. is serving macrobiotic food in its executive dining room

- In Peru, site of one of the largest coca leaf harvests in the world, a valley of farmers has stood up and said "no" to the drug lords and asked for macrobiotic assistance in developing an economy based on growing organic grains and vegetables

- In Russia medical doctors are using macrobiotic foods to help treat children and adults exposed to nuclear radiation because of the anti toxic effect of miso, sea vegetables and other macrobiotic quality foods

- In West Africa the macrobiotic community is actively distributing information on AIDS and diet and producing organic crops in an effort to overcome this dreadful scourge

Why this emphasis on macrobiotics? Because macrobiotics represents the deepest, most intuitive traditional wisdom of the human race, unifying people from all cultures and backgrounds. Along with other macrobiotic families around the world Mina, Bosko and their children invite you to become a part of this joyous, peaceful revolution. *My Beautiful Life* is an epic adventure, a book that will forever change your life.

Alex Jack
Becket, Massachusetts
February 7, 1998

Alex Jack teaches health care at the Kushi Institute and is director of the One Peaceful World Society in Massachusetts. He works closely with Michio Kushi and has co-authored several books with him. He is also author of several books including *Humanity at the Crossroads, The Mozart Effect, Inspector Ginkgo Tips His Hat to Sherlock Holmes* and *Profiles in Oriental Diagnosis.*

Introduction

The term "macrobiotic" was used in ancient Greece and comes from the root words "macro" originally meaning long or great and "bios" meaning life or living. It was found as far back as the fourth century B.C. in the writing of Hippocrates, the Father of Western Medicine. The term was used by other classical and Biblical writers to describe the importance of living in harmony with nature, eating a simple, balanced diet, and achieving a long, healthy life. In the Far East similar terms and concepts date back to the Yellow Emperor's *Classic of Internal Medicine*, the principal medical text of ancient China and the I Ching, the *Book of Changes*. The ideogram for peace in the Far East is composed of two characters representing "grain" and "mouth". Ancient people intuitively knew that eating whole cereal grains produced physical health and vitality; a calm, clear mind and sound judgement.

In the West the concept of macrobiotics continued through the Renaissance and enjoyed a brief resurgence of popularity in the 18th century. Dr. Christoph von Hufeland, a German medical doctor and physician to Goethe, published a book entitled *Macrobiotics, or the Art of Prolonging Life* in which he used new scientific discoveries and evidence such as the shape of the teeth and the length of the intestines, to support a return to a more traditional way of eating and lifestyle. In the East macrobiotics was reintroduced in the late 19th century by Sagen Ishizuki, M.D., a Tokyo based physician, who found that a diet centered on brown rice, miso, vegetables and sea vegetables could help prevent and relieve the infectious diseases which were then sweeping Japan and the rest of the industrialised world.

In the early twentieth century Yukikazu Sakurazawa (1893 – 1966) healed himself of advanced tuberculosis using Dr. Ishizuka's methods. Devoting his life to this method the young Japanese joined and became the leader of the small health food society of grateful patients, readers and associates of Dr. Ishizuka. In the late 20s and early 30s, Sakurazawa went to France to teach and write, and adopted George Ohsawa as his pen name. Later he revived the name "macrobiotics" to describe his teachings and he is now recognised as the Father of Modern Macrobiotics.

By the middle of the century traditional diets had virtually disappeared in both East and West, along with the understanding of using food as medicine. In the modern era new analytical methods of healing were the rule, and modern medicine moved from treating underlying causes of sickness and disease to relieving symptoms and effects.

Ohsawa taught that with proper diet we can have a great life full of adventure, freedom and endless joy and appreciation. He spent the better part of his life traveling and spreading macrobiotic principles and practices throughout the world including Southeast Asia, Africa, Europe and, towards the end of his life, North America. His students, most notably Michio and Aveline Kushi, who settled in the United States in the early 1950s, modified the diet to take into account different environmental and climatic conditions in the West as well as accommodate the needs of a modern lifestyle.

Over the last half century, the Kushis have served as the leaders of the international macrobiotic community. In the 1960s they launched the modern natural food movement so that whole grains; beans and bean products, including miso, tofu and tempeh; fresh, organically grown vegetables; sea vegetables and umeboshi plums, kuzu root and other medicinal plants were made available in natural foods stores across the United States and Europe. At first the medical profession ridiculed their teachings that modern diet was the underlying cause of heart disease, cancer and other degenerative disorders. But through seminars for medical professionals, scientific research at Harvard Medical School, the Framingham Heart Study and other research centers and most of all through case histories of ordinary people who recovered from serious illness with the help of macrobiotics, the Kushis initiated the diet and health revolution that today is changing the entire world.

By the early 1980s all of the major medical and scientific organizations issued dietary guidelines calling for substantial reductions in fatty foods as well as corresponding increases in whole grains, fresh vegetables and other minimally processed foods. In the early 1990s the U.S. government introduced the Food Guide Pyramid replacing meat and dairy food, the staples of the Four Food Groups, with a diet centered around grains, cereal products, fresh vegetables and fruit. While there are still some differences to be bridged, it is clear that the scientific and medical profession are moving in a macrobiotic direction. In 1995 a conference of several hundred medical researchers and nutritionists sponsored by the World Health Organization and Harvard University featured a macrobiotic banquet at the JFK Library in Boston with Michio Kushi as the guest of honor.

Today macrobiotic food is available at the Ritz Carlton Hotels around the world, at the international Prince Hotels, in an exclusive dining room at the Northwestern University business school and at numerous restaurants, schools, hospitals, nursing homes and other institutions. There is a Macrobiotic Society in the United Nations and, in 1994, Michio Kushi received the Award of Excellence from the UN Writers Society (awarded to the world's top authors) for his contribution to humanity. In 1999 the Smithsonian Institution will open a permanent Michio Kushi Family Collection on Macrobiotics and Alternative Health Care, featuring the Kushis personal papers, the literature of the natural foods and holistic health movements and an exhibition of cookware and foods. Either this year or next year the U.S. government will introduce national organic food standards for the first time, making better quality food widely available throughout the country.

As we enter the 21st century, the world is rediscovering whole, natural foods and moving towards a new model of health care. I am fortunate to have discovered this approach early long before it became popular. Not only did it save my life but it also broadened and deepened my understanding, providing a new direction and common bond for my family and myself. I have had the privilege of helping countless others to heal. This is the story of my life which led me to become a small part of this great health revolution.

Chapter 1

"The Year of Hope The Year of Salvation"

Roots of a Cherished Life

January 1987. Stara Pazova (formerly Yugoslavia). On page 10 of the number one nationally recognized magazine, "Illustrovana Politika", an article appears:

"Milenka Dobic, from Stara Pazova, is professor of linguistics and world literature and director of the Program of Radio Indjija. Looking younger than her 45 years she calmly and with clarity, tells us her story. An amazing story of all the happenings of her recent years' battle for life. It is succeeding! At last she can talk about it! Her face smiling and full of joy, she speaks of her husband, sixteen-year-old son and seven-year-old daughter. We are sitting with Milenka in her big, new, beautiful kitchen. Our eyes are fixed on the open pantry, abundant with labelled jars containing grains, beans, seaweed, dry mushrooms and foods with strange sounding Japanese names.

In that period of her life when she and her husband had just finished their life-time dream of building a new home; in those years when her children needed a mother's love more than ever (son a teenager, daughter just starting school); when her media career was at its peak, she had been told, "There is no hope for you. You have only two months to live!"

We are writing this story because we believe her testimony might help many people suffering from serious illnesses. For them this story could be the glimmer of light that guides them to discovering hope. Of course, some may say this is all fiction. But

Milenka Dobic's recovery cannot be explained any other way. Having been told that the remainder of her life would consist of aggressive therapy — namely radiation and chemotherapy — she turned her life around. She decided to make a radical break from the traditional approach to cancer and chose the macrobiotic way of life."

January 1997. Costa Mesa, California, U.S.A. Ten years have passed. I am reading about some woman diagnosed with Stage IV ovarian cancer and given two months to live. She chooses a strange new way of life and recovers within a year. Unbelievable! It's fiction! Yet strangely familiar...

Wake up, Mina! You are... I am that woman!! I was sentenced to death, as thousands of others before and after me have been, by the unanimous verdict of "scientific medicine." But a miracle intervened in the person of my medical doctor and best friend who knew about macrobiotics.

But how was such a rapid recovery possible? I was sick unto death. I felt it. The doctors said it. Yet today I am full of life, energetic, in radiant health, fulfilling all my dreams and sharing with others the strange secret that allowed nature to heal me.

In fact, it really isn't a secret. Every great traditional civilization knew the importance of living in balance — within yourself, with other people, with nature. Yet despite our space-age communications capabilities, it seems that we in the Western world have lost touch with this fundamental human concept. Around the planet others have healed, are healing, will heal from cancer... by the tens, hundreds, thousands. I'm writing this book for myself and others. It is my heartfelt wish that everyone could enjoy the same radiant health which the practice of macrobiotics has given me. I know now, even while safe in my mother's womb, that my destiny encompassed me, forcing me to search for a happy life. It took me almost half of my life to figure out that I am responsible for creating my own destiny. But I am getting ahead of myself. It all began...

Fifty-six years ago, in a little village northeast of Serbia in the Province of Vojvodina (in former Yugoslavia), I was the first-born child of Katrina and Kaja Popov. My mother, aided by a midwife, delivered me at home. I arrived in the middle of World War II — October 15th, 1942. It was that time of year when nature strung its most beautiful pearls. Trees were painted in brilliant hues of gold, red, burgundy, golden brown, splashed with reddish purple and turquoise.

Mother had post-birth complications and was unable to breast-feed. A Gypsy lady, my savior, breast-fed me until my mother was well enough to do it herself. I was a happy, healthy child. My father was off fighting the war for his people and country. My destiny has made me a fighter too!

Instead of sounds of a baby's toy rattle, my ears were learning to hear and enjoy the squeaking wheels of the wagons pregnant with autumn's harvest — from fields bursting with corn and sunflowers, from vineyards of grapes, from all the fields delivering their riches. I well remember mother's words, she said my tiny hands would quiver in the air when I heard a procession passing our house with the exquisite voices of the young harvesters anticipating celebration of the harvest festival.

Sadly that was the only singing I heard the first three years of my life. My mother never sang to me. Her heart was too heavy with loneliness because father was so far away, somewhere in the war with other family members.

Our village was a tiny citadel. We lived in tune with nature. Even those years of craziness and human destruction could not interrupt our traditional way of life.

That year autumn was most generous. Harvest-time was a traditional ritual. Each families' land was privately owned and cultivated during the year, but harvest-time became a communal affair. Field by field, nature yielded its gifts. All the neighbors, young and old, took part. That year we celebrated and prayed for war's end.

Once old enough, I participated in the harvest celebration. It was as if heaven and earth reverberated with young harvesters' voices. Women's aprons overflowed with grapes. Handsome baskets weighed down with all kinds of fresh vegetables and fruits, tables prepared with white tablecloths arranged with fresh picked food. After working tirelessly all day in the fields amongst autumn's fragrances, seventy or more people gathered. Laughing, singing, dancing, eating, full of joy, they mirrored the healthy food they had grown.

I close my eyes and relive that special time. I feel the goose bumps rise on my flesh. Vivid scenes of this traditional event linger fondly in my memory.

A gentle mantle of darkness falls upon our village. Fires burn on every street corner. Crowds pour into the wide streets. Even the elderly and ailing ones muster their strength and join the festivity. Celebrating continues long into the night.

Giant kettles of fresh salted popcorn overflow into waiting hands, permeating the night air with its hardy aroma.

The surrounding crowd bathes in its own sweat as it draws closer to the bonfire. Flaming tongues of fire lick the chilly autumn air, warming earth and sky. The contest begins. Half naked bodies of the older and braver get a running start. Lightning quick they leap over the flames. Fanning the fire as they jump scattering the huge sparks like sprinkles of fireworks. Night time resounds with screams and squeals mingled with delirious shouts of joy and laughter. Hats thrown high into the air. An enthusiastic throng cheers them on.

When the fire becomes exhausted the younger, braver children take turns hopping over the fire. Occasionally a shirt tail catches fire. On the opposite side of the flames their prize awaits. Friends shower them with a huge bucket of cooling water. Crowned winners are those doing it the most times. Streets boom with roaring applause.

Night is too short to contain the wellspring of emotions. The last bucket of water puts the crackling fires to sleep. Sunrise arrives too soon. Life is an exultation!

The celebration closes with prayers ascending with petitions for the safe return of our absent loved ones.

On August 21st 1945, our prayers were finally answered. The war ended. Father came home. That was one big happy day! In our village square the same people, wearing their traditional variety of national costumes, gathered again. Singing and dancing, deliriously happy, hugging loved ones — an emotional feast, fireworks in the heart — Odysseys of Peace!

There I was in mother's arms, feeling her warm tears on my cheek. My father caught sight of mother. She lifted me offering me up as a bouquet of fresh roses to our hero. I was three years old when my father and I first saw each other. Suddenly I disappeared into his huge overcoat. My cheek became blessed with his warm tears as he embraced me tightly. Without warning, a momentary wave of fear raced through my tiny body. I felt older than my three years as father, filled with pride, lifted me up for all the world to see — his badge of honor. That glorious day I first heard my parents singing. I sang too! The square became too small for the traditional welcoming celebration. Streets leading into the square were lined with tables. Red roses and fresh home-made breads adorned the white tablecloths. Red wine glistened in the glasses. A choir of voices resounded as one, toasting victory — Mir Zivileli! Peace — cheers! For my early childhood after years of war, this day was renaissance.

The following year we built a new home. A new member of our family arrived. Imagine my father's pride as he held his son in his arms. Now our family name would be carried on as our culture dictates. I watched father make the traditional public announcement of a male's birth. Standing in the moonlight, under a starlit sky, holding his hunting rifle above his head, he pointed it heavenward. In my little eyes he was larger than life. Ears covered, I watched him discharge a barrage of bullets and hurl his hat in the air. The announcement was now official. I'll never forget that very cold day, January 25th 1947 — two peaceful years after the war.

Like the trigger on a high-powered rifle, my mind flashes back to the day when my baby brother, Chedomir, was one year old. He had been diagnosed with polio, confined to a wheelchair with no hope of ever walking or running again. Mother was still very weak after childbirth, doing a few chores and then resting. But that evening, when my family gathered to decide what to do about my brother's illness, I saw her spirit stronger than ever.

My parents agreed on the course of action to be taken for his healing. Djurdjina, my maternal grandmother, was to take a major role in my brother's recovery. Doctors wouldn't allow mother in her weak condition, to stay in the hospital with my brother. So grandmother willingly volunteered to stay a month with him. His condition improved somewhat during that time but not as much as they hoped.

My grandmother and parents decided to bring him home. They chose to try traditional folk remedies, although this could be risky. The nearest city doctor was more than 20 miles away from our home.

There lived in our village a very old, long-time retired, Jewish doctor, affectionately called the *Medicine Doctor*. He recommended using healing clay from our pond; compresses made with wheat-bran and cabbage; herbal baths; and barley soup made with vegetables from our organic garden. And we loved Chedomir back to health.

My 6' 4" brother is now a healthy, strong, vibrant, 50 year-old man. Not only does he walk and run, he plays soccer, swims many miles, and rides his bike six kilometers daily. He's blessed with an adoring wife and two healthy children.

Although my brother recovered, mother didn't get any better. Despite this she was always there for us, loving us unconditionally. We didn't miss out on anything. We didn't realize until we were older how difficult it must have been for her. She sacrificed herself for our family's needs. If there had been trophies for "greatest mother," she would have gotten one.

Mother was a self-taught seamstress. She was more than that; she was an expert fashion designer. We never bought our own clothes. She designed beautiful dresses for herself and me and occasionally for other relatives. She made handsome suits and shirts for my father and brother. In fact she set the standard for fashion in our village. All the girls wanted to dress like me.

Visitors to our home were awed by mother's interior design and landscape artistry. A huge archway extended the full length of the walkway on the west side of the house. Twisting and turning, it culminated at the outside terrace in the back yard. Each side of the terrace was landscaped with an exquisite array of seasonal flowers with fragrances that made you feel as if you were in paradise. The full length of the archway was dressed with succulent grapes, in colors of burgundy, reddish purple, and white, each giving off its unique intoxicating aroma. Multicolored roses laced the walkway. What a breathtaking sight!

Set amidst that paradise was a table covered with a white cloth and embellished with picturesque dishes. There were always people at our home.

Mother's larger-than-life heart, warmer than sunshine smile, and engaging nature attracted everyone. And every day was a feast.

Mother worked from early morning to late at night. She went to the cornfields at 4 a.m. and worked all day and then returned to prepare dinner. Her culinary expertise was widely known. She was sought after and invited to supervise and oversee the most important events: weddings, christenings, and countless holiday celebrations.

Busy as she was, she always made time for her children. To teach us, and shape us into worthwhile individuals contributing to humanity. Daily she reminded us of the Golden Rule. In reverse! "Never do anything to someone you wouldn't want them to do to you." Her life's philosophy was natural and simple yet I felt sad. It seemed she lived her life only for us, leaving nothing over for herself. Whatever happened to us happened to her, too.

My teenage years were difficult for her. She dreamed of a prince charming who would snatch me away to a fairytale world, adored forever as his princess. For her a good life meant high recognition for women in society, with the respect accompanying that position.

My parents never argued or raised their voices in our presence. At no time was foul language heard in our home. Only once did I hear them discussing a major family problem regarding funding for our college education. Father calmly but sternly reminded her in no uncertain terms that he was and always would remain The Boss.

"Don't hit your head on the wall or knock yourself out. This is a man's decision! I'll handle it my way. Go back to the kitchen. Stay in your place. Take care of the children and house, and leave the rest to me." Period!

She knew what "his way" meant. It would take an eternity to accumulate enough money. And it would only be for my brother's education. After all "… a woman's place is in the kitchen" and that's where I belonged, too. Mother didn't argue. She knew that even if she won the battle she'd lose the war. But she got her way. Brilliantly she devised a plan to safeguard her self-worth, and free *me* from the kitchen.

Actually, what she did was outside the accepted moral framework of our society. To raise funds needed for both children's college education, she gambled her own reputation. What others thought didn't deter her. Nothing stopped her. Her resolve was unshakable!

She opened the doors of her home to earn money for her children's college education. She did this by serving meals. Well-meaning, conservative thinkers criticized her for allowing "perfect strangers" into her home, especially while her husband was away.

Her comment was: "You know your life, I know mine. Thank you for your concern." She knew she was benefiting her family and the people she was serving. Among her customers were the intellectual elite of the community, male and female. Doctors, engineers, managers, and teachers. This gave her an opportunity to display her artistry to an appreciative audience. The food, its presentation and her hospitality made for an enchanting gathering. Affectionately they called her *Mother Katarina*.

One day a gentlemen customer surprised her with a beautiful bouquet of red roses. Touched by his gesture of kindness she felt appreciated and acknowledged for the first time as a woman and a human being. It was as if a rose had brushed her cheeks, leaving behind its color. She radiated a beauty that made the roses blush with embarrassment and bow shyly in her presence. Her eyes sparkled with a new brightness and she took on a glow reminiscent of her youth.

Sadly, father never made her feel that way. Yet I knew he loved her in his own way. As I grew older I urged him to pay more attention to her. His response was always the same.

"Mind your own business. I have better things to do than play in your comedy." I never stopped trying, and he never changed.

It was morally embarrassing in my parents' time to openly express emotions in front of others. Mother, more willing to take a risk, laid bare her emotions. Father never dared. So that playful, whimsical, and uninhibited husband-wife relationship suffered as a result.

She set about to fill that void by surrounding herself with reflections of love. Realizing there was little opportunity for young people to spend time together and express their feelings toward each other she opened our home to them. At that time girls were not allowed to go out alone. They were chaperoned at all times. If there was a dance, mothers always accompanied their daughters to and from the dance.

Many a cold winter evening when I was a child, the youth gathered at our home. We cherished those loving, enchanting times. They rushed to our home, full of energy, ready to explore life's wondrous adventures. A feast awaited them. Tables were arranged with snacks and home-made pastries. They played parlor games. But other things were going on under the table. That was my favorite place to spy on them.

Quietly and in hiding, I watched mother. As the young girls' angelic voices rose in song, tears of pearls like early morning dew moistened her crocheting. Her deep-seated emotions smothered, her life was bereft of excitement. The ashes, leftovers, crumbs, the scraps, and sediment of a loveless life were buried deep in her chest. The outcome — tuberculosis, from which she never recovered.

From the time I was old enough to remember, I was constantly at her side. Her face was radiant as she taught me. It was joyful. My fondest desire was to be exactly like her. She was my ideal. I adored her and I was proud to be her daughter. As for father, we saw him only on weekends. He was employed by the sugar factory to negotiate contracts with private farmers for their sugar beets, so much of his time was spent travelling to various villages. He was a very loving father. My brother and I were always competing for his "lap space" and most of the time I lost.

At sixteen, I rose at four in the morning and ran to the station. The train took me the six miles into the city to attend high school. I was away from home all day long and returned about 4 p.m. For lunch I took along a sandwich, smothered with lard, salt and cayenne pepper but was often too busy to eat it. Kids who could afford it ate cheese pies. Sometimes, if Grandpa gave me a little money, I treated myself to cheese pie too. I was a good daughter. I never complained. I got so much love at home other things faded into insignificance.

My parents lived and reared us by a strict moral code. We willingly obeyed and in no way were we ever abused. At eighteen, I still had to ask father's permission to go picnicking, see a movie, or even go to a girl friend's house to do homework. That's the way all of us were reared in my generation. And none of us ever felt deprived.

Father was a man with high ideals. His ideology meant doing whatever his country called upon him to do. By so doing, he believed he served not only his country, but family and others as well. He joined the cause of the people for all the right reasons. Willingly sacrificing everything on behalf of the

Communist ideology, he brought peace to others, but found none for himself. His deepest disappointment was seeing the blatant hypocrisy of the Communist leaders. The war won, they greedily took the spoils for themselves, breaking their promises of equality for all. Hurt and enraged at the same time, father broke all ties with the system that betrayed him. He threw his party membership card in the faces of the cheaters, severing the umbilical cord forever.

Gratifying as that was, we all paid a high price. Covertly we were black-listed. Both my brother and I were denied scholarships. Father and I went to his wartime buddy, Jovan, an official high in the state hierarchy, to request help in finding jobs for my brother and me. What a sad commentary on history that two highly educated and over-qualified citizens couldn't get a job. This was the more remarkable in view of the fact that priority for scholarships and jobs were given to children of wartime veterans. That is, for everybody — except father.

The scenario of that visit went something like this. We walked through the sound-proof doors overlaid with rich, stuffed burgundy leather. We saw a man sitting in his high-back leather chair with a life-size wall hanging of President Tito on the left and one of Lenin adorning the wall on the right. There he sat, behind his huge mahogany desk, wearing a designer suit, with a tie the color of our flag.

"Hello Jovan. Are you the same man that I shared my last piece of cornbread with at the Igman Odyessy?" father asks with just a hint of sarcasm.

"Time passes by, we are getting older. Don't you recognize me?"

"I'm not talking about your age, I'm talking about your affluence."

"What can I do for you?" Jovan responds coldly.

"Maybe you can tell me why my children can't get work. They are both highly qualified. As you well know, our friends' kids, who are much younger and less qualified, all got good jobs years ago." Father's right hand automatically motions toward his chest as he places his hand under his medal of honor, his head slightly bowed. With this gesture, the real question being silently asked is: "Is it possible to erase the patriot who was willing to unconditionally surrender his life on behalf of his countrymen?" Instead, struggling to keep his patience, father politely fashions the question, lowering his voice, "Am I black-listed, Comrade?"

Jovan leaps up from his chair. His left fist pounds on the desk as his body leans forward. Like an arrow finding its target, his right index finger points its warning in the face of his "wartime buddy." The droplets of perspiration collecting on his forehead and his beet-red face betray his intense, barely controlled anger.

He heartlessly shouts, "I don't know what you are talking about. Maybe your children didn't look hard enough or maybe they're expecting more than they deserve."

"O.K.", said father. "I see there is nothing for me here. I came to the wrong place and the wrong person. I think there is no right place and no right person for me. Do you really think we were fighting for that? One million seven hundred thousand of our countryman died — for what? Nothing's changed. Kurta sjashi and Murta uzjashi!" (This expression means: Kurta mounts the horse and Murta, who is really Kurta being called by a different name, dismounts the horse.)

Each successive heartbeat chokes Jovan as he gazes malevolently at father. He shouts the words like a snapping shark, "Don't you realize that people are imprisoned for saying less than that? But because you're my friend I will overlook it... this time."

Father feels a perilous necessity to speak. As they lock contact, eye to eye, he comes to the end of his patience, "Don't you ever call me that again. I'm not your friend."

And with one quick, sweeping movement, he turns his back and walks away from his past.

That stressful event proved to be the major turning point for our whole family. My brother and I came to the realization that we had to do everything for ourselves. He stayed home with father, as was the custom, waiting for a job and a place at law school. To support my studies I had taken a job. Now I had to move closer to my work. That was the most painful decision of my life since mother was gravely ill.

Mother and father lived for the two of us. They invested all their savings in our education. And we made them proud of us. At the age of 23 I got my masters degree in linguistics and world literature and began to teach while working on my doctorate.

Mother passed away on March 9th 1969, three days before her forty-fifth birthday. She wanted me to be a teacher and I was determined to be the best. I achieved all the awards an educator could be given. If only she had lived long enough to see all her dreams come true!

The saddest day of my life was when mother died in my arms. Her last words were: "You're my sunshine." It was her final blessing to me. I accepted her last words as my commitment. For me it meant to be a light and to give light everywhere.

While my brother was attending law school, I worked two jobs to support him. Weekends I travelled home 36 miles to help my father and brother keep house. I tried my best to keep mother's spirit alive. I married in 1971 and in 1977 so did my brother. He and his wife Zlata lived with our father, who had never remarried. He helped to rear their family and was the best teacher, baby sitter, diaper changer. And for all the love he gave, he got even more in return.

Periods of long separation from mother had taken its toll on father. So much of her short life was spent in sanatoriums. When she finally died his life no longer had the same meaning. He had lost the love of his life and bore that pain twenty five years.

A friend reminded me that the Bible says, "We plant the seed and we water it, but God's love makes it grow." I remember mother teaching me the same thing. As we collected the beans in our garden I can still hear her saying, "From just one bean, thousands will come. Don't waste them." Later in my life I again saw the wisdom in that. Indeed, I was yet to learn the profound meaning of "from one grain, a thousand grains." My life looked to me like a field under cultivation, sowing seeds and reaping the harvest.

Chapter 2
Loving What I Do

A new era of my life began when I moved far away from my parents' home. I got a job as professor of literature and linguistics in Sremski Karlovci, which is a little town in the southwest of Vojvodina Province and the hub of activity there.

I was fortunate to get this job and determined to gain approval for who I was, and not be judged by my family history. Grateful for my creative spirit, I resolved to set a precedent in teaching, changing its face, and contributing generously to human relationships.

A few of us dared strike out in new directions. "What is the Name of Your School?" I asked. "What Have You Done for Your Community?" These questions became the foundation for the first community service program for students in grades four through twelve. They worked to see who could provide the greatest service to their community.

For example, students helped elderly people in their homes; ran errands, cleaned, and assisted in maintaining their property. They cleaned and cared for parks, streets, schools, factories, and businesses. At harvest-time thousands of students joined the community working side by side with farmers to bring in crops. They weren't alone. Teachers, and sometimes parents, worked alongside them. For this they accrued credits which they exchanged for things the schools needed, such as computers, movie and slide projectors and other teaching equipment. This program was such a success it served as the model later adopted by the entire country!

This program was broadcast on radio. As each student completed assigned tasks she/he phoned the radio station and was patched in live to the program. The audience evaluated the student's work.

Another innovative teaching assignment was applied in literature. It was a team effort in which each student had the freedom to create. A typical assignment might be: do an analysis of the famous novelist, Pearl Buck. The class was divided into smaller groups of four or five students, each given one month to prepare and report on specific aspects of the assignment. For example: Group 1: Historical viewpoint; Group 2: Geographical location given in detail; Group 3: Present theme of the novel; Group 4: Characterizations of each person in the novel; Group 5: Language and grammar. We didn't confine our classes to within a building; we took them outside to share in nature. The young people were ablaze with excitement, like worker bees busily occupied in caring for their beehive. Among students with previously low grade averages, a metamorphosis gushed within as they discovered their real potential. Everyone got an opportunity to express himself. Not one student received a failing grade! Three years in a row my classes won Literary Awards for recitation of poetry and original writing.

In those classes where the teachers didn't participate, students tended to repeat classes and do make up work through summer break. Later, more teachers participated in the program, and their results were similar to mine. In all my 30 years of teaching, never once did any student repeat a grade. Why? Because time was never an issue. I gave each one of them all the time they needed to develop their skills and integrity. The goal was to build intellectual strength and a personal level of security, so they were no longer dependent on the teacher. We worked together until they got it right. My reward was watching this crowd of youth searching out the deeper meaning of knowledge, grateful and satisfied for their discovery.

Because of pressure, it's difficult for teachers to remember their real mission. Is it not the mission of teachers to prepare future generations to apply theoretical knowledge in their practical life? School is the place to gather knowledge but, unfortunately, most students don't use it until they grow up. That's the problem. Whereas, if they use what they learn immediately, both they and society benefit right away. And that is the solution to the problem. Then it becomes easier for young people to find an important place in society and contribute to its development.

At the time I was teaching, the educational system was stagnating from lack of funds in a very poor country. As you might expect, educators were poorly paid. So there was very little incentive for them to do anything creative other than what the curriculum dictated. A few young enthusiasts were trying hard to stir up that dead sea of mediocrity. We strove with all the enthusiasm we could muster to make changes. And it wasn't easy. We had plenty of opposition. Teachers' attitudes were also a factor. Veteran teachers tended to ask, "Why should we do that? We aren't paid for it."

In contrast, my friends and I believed it necessary to see the whole picture, understanding that it's not all about money. We need to invest in our children. They are our future. However, only a few of us were striving for change. The majority were content to preserve the status quo.

Yet I'm happy to say that the changes we initiated, which started as an experiment, caught the attention of the entire educational system. Because of their success they were later incorporated into the curriculum. For something like this to work you must have the right teacher. The teacher has to have love. The teacher has to love what he or she is doing. She must be an innovator. A magnet for students, so school becomes the place where they long to be.

I believe I was born to be a teacher. Teaching… it felt like being on stage and my students were right on stage with me. I had so much appreciation for them. All of us thoroughly enjoyed that stimulating, creative, educational experience. Each class was like attending a premier. It wasn't teacher and student, it was a premier performance! I loved my work, I loved what I did. I poured my soul into it.

My students loved me and I loved them with all my heart. As if holding a delicate flower carefully, we were absorbed in a learning process, laughing excitedly, talking, ignoring the school bell. Nobody wanted to leave the classroom. We all wanted this to last forever. I was privileged to leave an indelible mark on the educational system. And I will never stop teaching. How could I? After all, life is learning and teaching. The two are inseparable.

But that especially stressful period in my life contributed to high blood pressure, kidney problems and insomnia. After I had been on medication for these a couple of years, next appeared asthma and allergies. Twice a week for ten years I took allergy shots. I didn't get better. I got worse!

When I was working long hours, I didn't make time to eat. If I did, it was only to satisfy hunger. Foods I could chew fast and swallow fast. Almost immediately my body would react. And I'd say to myself, "I shouldn't have eaten that." But that didn't stop me from eating that same food again and again, in spite of the adverse reaction.

I asked my friends, doctors Andria and Ratka Rudic, for medical advice. My body responded instantly to the medication. Relief was immediate but temporary. Symptoms reappeared. I got the feeling there's no real cure for me. I'd just have to live with it.

For years I had been on kidney medication. While I was hospitalized for a severe kidney attack, the doctor told me that my inflamed tonsils were causing kidney problems. He urged their removal, assuring me my health would improve. So at 26 I heeded his advice. Shortly thereafter I began having serious multiple allergies. In springtime I got shots every two weeks for pollen, dust and nicotine.

While I was suffering with high blood pressure, no one ever suggested I change my diet, except to stop eating saturated fats. My doctor kept repeating the same thing, "Try this medication. If this doesn't work, we'll try something else." I trusted him implicitly. Why wouldn't I? I didn't know anything about Western medicine or how to treat my illness.

I didn't know enough to ask him about possible side effects. And I certainly had my share of them. Sometimes the side effects were worse than my illness.

My overall health condition worsened when I decided to change my career and enter the media world. In 1976, I became Director of Education, Arts and Entertainment for Radio Indjija. It is one of the most popular local stations in that region, in fact in the whole Province of Vojvodina. I held that position for eleven years. That period of my life was possibly the most stressful. In 1986, I accepted the added responsibility of creating and directing the Special Educational Programming at Radio Belgrade.

At the same time, from 1982 to 1987, I did freelance writing for daily and weekly newspapers, contributing articles of interest to all educational levels, from preschool to university. I traveled regularly within the province, serving as a representative at meetings of various Boards for about twelve different local radio stations. I organized the first Radio School of Journalism for Youth. Special youth programs were established for each level: elementary, high school and university. Each school appointed students as reporters and journalists. They participated in a competition by broadcasting their reports on the radio. Radio Indjija liked my idea and ran with it.

We enlisted the local business owners, large corporations, state organizations, agricultural unions, and state-owned factories to contribute much needed funds and equipment to the award-winning schools. This live radio talk show program became very popular. It was one of the programs most listened to, and the phone lines were jammed with listeners anxious to participate in the live broadcast.

In 1985 I expanded my career to include writing, directing and producing documentaries on current issues for TV Novi Sad's Arts and Entertainment Program. During my eleven year media career I received many awards for journalism. One of the most coveted awards in Yugoslav journalism is the "Truth" award. I was privileged to receive this in 1986 as writer/producer/director of a comprehensive documentary entitled "One Step from Death to Life" devoted to survivors of the Holocaust.

Because of my work with youth and students, I was offered sole responsibility for creating, producing, and directing a huge production. It was for our national Youth Day Holiday, May 25th 1986. This meant coordinating three thousand students and some fifty soldiers. The event was held in the biggest football stadium in our province. The theme of the production was an introduction to the history of our country. It was arranged as a series of scenes or individual vignettes, set to music and poetry.

The choreographic presentation included ballet, modern dance and acrobatic creations. The students were assigned to wear various colored costumes. Each side of their costumes were a different color. They were strategically positioned in the stadium. On cue they stood in unison. As if guided by an invisible hand, turning from left to right, their bodies spelled out the words: *Brotherhood, Unity, Peace* and *Happy Youth Day.*

Each scene was delivered with precision and grace. As they turned to the left, six torches took shape representing each of the six republics. As they turned to the right, they formed a blazing sun that quickly coalesced into stars. Finally they formed our country's vibrantly colored flag.

The climax was the most picturesque of all — a tribute to our idol, our President. The audience was awestruck as they silently read each letter which formed the words: *Salute! Tito! Happy Birthday!* Then as the students moved their bodies forward and swayed from side to side an exquisite bouquet of red roses appeared, moving this way and that, as if touched by a gentle spring breeze. It was breathtaking. It was heart-stopping. The participants and the audience created the finale by rising in thunderous applause!

Typically, I started rehearsals for this show in early Spring. Nature was waking up, attention-evoking fragrances overtook the smog, everything was blooming — and so were my allergies! No wonder, because I was always too busy to eat. When I did finally take a quick snack it was usually my "proven pressure relievers"… yogurt and pastries. After that I would feel much worse and become afraid to eat. Sometimes I didn't eat anything all day. I forgot to eat.

My body was experiencing the boundless energy that only youth possesses, believing it would always be the same. The playful spirit and contagious joyfulness of the students filled my soul. We made a deal. Usually teachers are addressed as *Professor.* Mina, in my Serbo Croatian language, means "a mine" (bomb). When the crowd got so loud and drowned out my instructions, they shrieked with laughter, jokingly saying, "You'd better be quiet, or you will activate the "mine."

I wished this connection would never end. Their effervescence, spontaneity and inner intensity spilled over into everything they did. We lived in the warm, invisible light of friendship, laboring together toward a common goal. I needed no further assurance: the price I was paying wasn't too high. Yet in that moment, bursting with youthful spirit, what a picture I was: puffy face, tearful, blurry eyes, runny nose, pounding ears, congested lungs, barely able to breathe. I was suffering and struggling with script and tissues in one hand, megaphone in the other, pockets bulging with dozens of prescription drugs, multiple inhalers (just in case I ran out of the first two, I always had one or two more for backup). I was running out of hands. But I never missed a day. I was always there.

By the end of the third month I was physically exhausted — a basket case! The show was a smashing success. I cried, they cried and the hugging was endless. We celebrated together until the early morning and allowed the rising sun to glorify the moment.

Chapter 3

Private Bliss
and Disappointment

My professional life had been a triumphant progress, my personal life a series of peaks and lows. I was so busy working, I had very little time for building relationships. Besides in my culture females, especially teachers, had to be circumspect, above reproach, almost saints. If a teacher were to become a member of the Communist Party, worse still. Her morality had to be nun-like. In short, I had no close private life until I married Bosko. I met him in 1970 about one year after my mother died. The timing couldn't have been better. God sent him to me just when I needed him most.

At the time I appeared to be in good shape physically, mentally, and spiritually, but inside I was rotting away. Meeting Bosko happened like this. My very good friend Rushka taught English at the same school I did. Bata was Rushka's boyfriend. His best friend was Bosko. Bata's car was in the body shop and he asked Bosko to drop him off at my apartment.

At that time I was one of the very few people who owned a TV. I had invited friends over to watch the Olympics. Into my apartment and into my life walked this young, tall, handsome, intelligent, and very funny student, Bosko Dobic. He was studying International Business at the University of Economics in the capital city of Belgrade. From the first moment our eyes met, the chemistry was explosive. The next day we went on a picnic, and, as they say, the rest is history.

When we met, he was in a two-year relationship and I was practically engaged to someone else. At first, I didn't tell anybody about him because he was a "younger" man. I was his senior by three-and-a-half years. When I finally confided my intentions to my best friend, who was born in Stara Pazova, the same village as Bosko's mother, she begged me, "Please don't marry him if you have to live together with his mother!" Love is blind.

I married my husband, but I also married his mother. The first month I tasted the bitter fruit of my friend's advice. My mother-in-law was a very jealous and controlling person. To whatever I said, she added her distorted thinking. She took pleasure in deliberately twisting the meaning of my words in order to demean me.

I felt worthless. I can't describe my frustration. Inside me burned a compelling desire to use all my potential, the last ounce of energy to vindicate myself. As if in a vice, inch by unbearable inch, my life force was being slowly squeezed out of me. In a vain attempt to escape my misery, I made the pursuit of materialism my goal. I reasoned that by putting all my energy into my work I could somehow evade the emptiness I felt in the depths of my soul.

Sadly, my poor husband was a tortured man. He tried to stand up for me at no small cost to himself. He was his mother's only child. Within him a battle raged between a mother he loved and honored and a wife he desperately cherished. He didn't want to hurt her. But he didn't know how to defend himself. His mother was uneducated. Perhaps this was the only way she knew to express herself. So he excused her rather than accusing her. It was easier to surrender than to take a firm stand. Bosko had adopted this strategy early on in order to survive.

The thought did occur to me to leave. But just as quickly I dismissed that option. To do so would humiliate my family. Our culture and its moral code were uncompromisingly strict. A divorced woman was looked down upon. Especially a teacher if reared in a conservative household. Moreover, I loved Bosko. The sparks of our love ignited our souls, setting the stars on fire.

By staying I paid a very high price. The first years of my marriage, I had total financial responsibility for the household. Bosko was still completing his studies. My mother-in-law had never worked. The second year of my marriage I got pregnant. Then there was absolutely no turning back.

My pregnancy was the most exciting and beautiful moment in our marriage. But not for my mother-in-law! My husband and I got closer. Her unpleasantness got worse. On May 25th 1972, Youth Day and President Tito's birthday, our son Srdjan was born. I felt like I had just received a very special award. I nursed him for fifteen months. In the fourteenth month he started to develop respiratory problems. We couldn't fully enjoy rearing our son because we were constantly under attack from Srdjan's grandmother. I believed then and believe now that stress was transported through my milk into our child's body.

Today I see things differently. I couldn't have done any better because I didn't know any better. I was blind to the truth that I had created the situation myself, allowing it to happen by the choices I made. All my life I had tried to please others. I could break the fetters of conservatism in my career, but was never able to achieve a better quality of personal life. I never loved myself enough to be able to defend myself. I had forfeited my chance to be my own hero. Possessing everything a woman could want — a man I adored, a beautiful son, wonderful friends, great career. I was a strong person, powerful, yet something inside me was hollow. Something essential was missing. I couldn't find enough passion to fill up that hole in my soul, to direct my destiny in the right way.

On the one hand I felt worthless, undefined. On the other I was still empowered with unlimited energy to achieve, to do, to go. One part of me wanted to reach for the sky in the professional world. Another part of me — my inner self, my feminine and motherly self — strove to nurture my family and keep the fires of my family hearth burning. I lived crucified like that for four full years. Our little family had its best times when we were away from home. Our love kept me going and surviving all the emotional barricades. It was a glorious flag announcing our victory.

Somehow all my life I expected only crumbs of happiness. Never put myself first in any situation or established relationship. Always I was carried by the tide of other people's feelings and desires.

Somehow I had not connected with my deeper self. Instead I lived out my emotional turmoil lamenting my destiny. I played the victim. Now I see clearly that nobody was to be blamed for anything. I chose that path myself. I'm amazed when I think about all my complicated, dramatic, romantic, remorseful attempts to reach happiness. I never got there.

At the age of nineteen-and-a-half I had left my parents' home. As a teacher in a little Srem village, I was obsessed more with my image than my real feelings. These moral shackles were the foundation of my upbringing. My mother was always proud of me. When she was swept away by tuberculosis, leaving forever behind her the burdens of this earth, I lost half of myself and remained perplexed.

So my emotional life was still muffled at that time. I kept smothering all my love flames, ignoring their importance in the life of a young woman. My biggest worry was "What would others think of me?" It was not only created by the humdrum atmosphere of the village I lived in, it was also the pattern of my strict, traditional upbringing that almost became the core of my social code.

The religious background of my mother's family shackled me with moral dogmas for life. I see now how stressful that was. I prefer to say I was living up to the expectations of others. Even my marriage required me to sacrifice. Love for my husband had to be muffled to avoid conflict with my mother-in-law's "love" feelings for her only son. Again and again I backed down, suffering, my life energy dribbling into an abyss. I sentenced myself to burn withdrawn in the flames of my enormous love for my husband. I was choking with repressed love, not taking hold of the advantages and privileges of the most beautiful challenge which confronts a young woman. I was crucified between my normal sensuous being and the world of dark sensual powers. I loved and suffered, punishing myself without reason.

Many times Bosko and I ran from that hell to find out what real love is. We stayed together, sometimes happy, but the scars were getting deeper and deeper. Emotional chaos, problems at home and work, were burning me out.

Our first-born Srdjan was caught in that frustrated family atmosphere. Bosko loved him to the sky. But when Srdjan was three months old, the head of our family, my love, my husband, was drafted into the reserve army.

All of a sudden, I had to support three of us on my modest teacher's salary — my son, myself and my mother-in-law. She was in very good physical condition but never used her energy to help me through those hardships. I rushed between home and work, frustrated with my life, exhausted by the bizarre circumstances that enfolded my everyday reality. Then one day I couldn't take it any more. I packed two bags of clothes for my son and myself and went to live in Indjija.

It was very hard. Living alone in a rented place. Shuttling the baby back and forth to his sitter. Running to school to lecture and back again to care for my child. What a stress-filled life. Watch my diet? I never did. I ate what was there. It was only important for my baby to have fresh food.

Fifteen months later, Bosko returned. Not long after, he got a well paid factory job. We moved into a beautiful house. Lived by ourselves and rediscovered a powerful love. We laughed, sang, and enjoyed life for the very first time. *Pax tandem* — peace at last!

Those were the best years. A veritable renaissance of our marriage. We lived in a dream world. My allergies improved. I cooked for my family. My way, using lots of vegetables. Before my mother-in- law had been the cook so we ate excess fat, meat, dairy and baked flour products. Now I was free. I changed all that.

Regretfully, our bliss didn't last long. My mother-in-law begged, pleaded, wept. She broke Bosko's heart. Reluctantly we agreed to return to her home in Stara Pazova. We cut a deal. Bosko's name was added to the deed. The house was renovated. Our family got private quarters. It became our love nest... for a while.

First Srdjan developed bad allergies. Mine came next. We became steady hospital visitors. Each getting our allergy shots twice a week. Again my mother-in-law invaded our private quarters. While I worked she came, demeaning me in Bosko's and Srdjan's eyes. Again life was hell. I developed high blood pressure, bad allergies, lumps on my legs, cysts on my ovaries. I was to be on medication for ten years, my condition never improving. Old cysts vanished, new ones took their place. I was grievously unhappy. Western medicine wasn't helping me. My personal life was a shambles. My only joys were my son and my husband... when mother-in-law wasn't around. For me there was no exit.

Then one serendipitous idea saved us all! We decided to build our own home. After living in the Stara Pazova house seven years, we rented a house near my work in Indjija. We built a new one-bedroom house in my mother-in-law's back yard. She moved in. We tore down the old moldy, unhappy house. On that spot we built a tri-level, six bedroom, three bathroom, 3,000 square foot home. It was exquisite!

This building project could have been stressful. Instead it was a delightful experience. In part due to Yelena's birth. She arrived by "special request" of her brother. What a happy and healthy child! And the whole family was living in a wholesome environment.

In 1985, we moved into our new home in Stara Pazova. Peace was made with my mother-in-law. Fifteen years had passed. No longer could she say those cutting words, "This is my house." Remembering that trauma made me cringe. Today, with my new life perspective, her comment is laughable.

We had built our material world. And satisfied the middle class social standard we'd created for ourselves. Finally we thought we had it all. We had made peace with the past. We weren't worried about the future. That's because illness was forcing us to deal with the present.

Our son suffered chronic asthma. He survived by using medication and inhalers. As for me I gained weight, had migraines, allergy attacks, kidney problems, incredibly painful PMS. Yelena had hernia surgery at age four. At age five we noticed a recurrence of the same symptoms on the opposite side. Bosko had been suffering for years from digestive disorders and bleeding hemorrhoids. We were all victims of our lifestyle and diet. We couldn't change that. We didn't know how. Medication prescribed by Western medicine was our only hope. And that wasn't working.

In early 1986 my health was in shambles. I spent the entire year going from one specialist to another, searching for medical solutions for chronic fatigue and other related problems. By May I was in a state of crisis.

My health was on a greased, down-hill runway headed toward a stone wall. I was suffering excruciating and repetitious migraines, pressure on the top of my head, vertigo, fast declining energy level, appetite loss and depression. I was also diagnosed with nephritis of the kidneys.

These multiple symptoms prompted my physician to initiate a series of tests. They came back negative. They told us nothing. Our best friend Andrija Rudich, M.D., expedited my appointments. In the next month-and-a-half I had a series of x-ray exams: lungs, gall bladder, colon, and brain. My entire body was saturated with radiation. My body kept sounding the alarm. Blood pressure soared off the charts. Joints were swollen. Rectal pressure was so intense I couldn't sit, stand, or sleep. Each step was pure torture. I was disintegrating.

Scariest of all was loss of memory. My position at the radio station required a person to be able to sustain high energy levels, sharp thinking, self sufficiency. These qualities and abilities were slipping away. What was wrong?

Reviewing the battery of tests, the specialist concluded: "Early menopause!" So they assigned me to a drug marathon. The doctors systematically divided my body into compartments. For each compartment they prescribed a different medication. Any one could have made me an addict. No one looked at my body as a whole, coordinated prescribed dosages or considered systemic side effects. Fortunately my body knew what to do. Two days after consuming the drugs I collapsed on the bus. I awoke in Andrija's office.

As he stood over me he asked, "Mina, you smell like a pharmacy. What did you take?"

My tongue was thick and heavy, my mouth dry and parched. I struggled to get the words out, "They're in my purse." My voice tended to disappear. I didn't see his reaction but I heard his words.

"How many did you take today?"

"Please, check what I wrote on the memo pad."

"My God! Why did you take six different drugs in the morning?"

"I don't know. I'm just sick of you doctors. Throw away all those drugs."

My dear husband came immediately, aware at once of the urgency. He embraced me, tears streaming down his face.

"What happened to you?" Sensing the crisis, he wheeled around to our friend. "Andrija, is there any way you can help Mina?"

I answered instead of Andrija. "I think it's too late. I believe I have cancer."

Bosko was terrified. "What are you talking about?"

"I'm talking about how I feel. Take me home."

Andrija didn't say anything. But after his shift was over he came to see me. He suggested I see a gynecologist. Instead I went back to work, saying nothing to anyone. To sit was unbearably painful. When no one was around I stood up to type in a futile attempt to relieve the pain. If anybody entered my office I had to sit but would keep shifting my weight from one side of my bottom to the other. Meanwhile, some strange voice was confirming my greatest fear: "You have cancer."

Then, suddenly, during an interview, the person, the room, everything in it, started spinning out of control. I collapsed. Bosko came quickly and took me to my gynecologist. He couldn't do an examination. I was in too much pain to let him touch me. He called his best friend at the major hospital in the province. A few minutes later I became their patient. That was the last time my children saw me for twenty two days.

At that time I didn't realize the full impact of my illness on my family. Eleven years later I learned how much my absence affected my six-year-old daughter. Quite by accident, I overheard a conversation between Yelena and her friend. She told a story I'd never heard before.

"I was too young to be allowed to visit Mom in the hospital, so I set up my own vigil each night, cuddling up with my blanket at our front door. I didn't want to watch TV. I didn't want to sleep in my own bed. I was waiting for Mommy to come home. As soon as I fell asleep Daddy and big brother carried me upstairs to my bedroom. This went on for about a month, until Mommy finally came back home."

For me hospital was prison. I was confined to a bed. No more blue sky, singing birds, sunshine, fresh air — only monotony. All day long I heard the complaints of my room-mates. Every two hours, a medical technician took me for an examination, handed me medication, supervised my every move.

Horror of horrors, gynecological examinations were performed by medical students needing practice! Sometimes, twice a day. One day the head surgeon, a gynecologist, and two students examined me. The doctor explained my symptoms. Then directed each student in turn as he performed the gynecological procedure. I cried in pain and begged them to stop.

"What's the matter? Do you want to be helped or not?" the head surgeon screamed at me, with a martyred expression.

Tearfully I answered him, my voice escalating to hysteria, "Isn't one examination enough? I can't stand the pain. Let me go!"

Even more arrogantly, he shouted, nostrils flaring, "I know what is enough. You can go now."

The pain in my chest was like an arrow being pulled from a deep wound. I felt weak and broken. I was barren and empty. My femininity was raped.

I was a quivering tangle of mixed feelings; part overwhelming disappointment, part smoldering anger. I was wrenched and shattered.

Frail as I was, I struggled to get to my room, leaving a trail of blood marking my way. I asked a nurse passing in the hallway for something to stop the bleeding. Turning around, I came face to face with that doctor. He swaggered toward me, wearing the same pious look, overflowing with unsociable remoteness. I bet he was born on the unfriendly side of a valley.

"Doctor, that last exam left me with even more pain. I'm bleeding," I complained, irritated by his loftiness.

He cleared his throat and demanded with a superior air, "What are you doing in the hallway when you're bleeding? Why aren't you in bed?"

"I'm looking for help," I blurted out.

"Go to bed and wait for the nurse to come," was his pitiless command.

I gazed bewildered at this bullet-headed man, conscious of his grim mood. I had no intention of shrinking away defencelessly. I boiled over with a roar.

"Is that all you can say? Isn't it enough you make me feel guilty, as if I'm breaking hospital rules. Well, let me tell you, you break human rules. Where is your ethic? The way you treat patients is disgusting, degrading, and inhuman. Don't you recognize me? I'm a journalist and human rights advocate. I suggest you get a haircut, so you'll look good on TV. Perhaps you'd like to tell my TV colleagues how you treat your patients. And then we'll interview your patients. That will make a great headline on the evening news."

As I relive this episode of my life, I feel embarrassed to admit my attitude, because doctors are also human beings and they have their good and bad days. I assume they have good intentions, doing the best they know how to help sick people. The person who attacked him was not the person I am inside. It was out of character for me to judge anyone harshly. My illness was talking. My anger propelled by fear.

He passed by me undaunted. The next day he didn't show up. I was summoned to the medical office. When I walked in I saw a different doctor and another group of students. I prepared to forestall them.

"Oh, no. This is not going to happen again. No more examinations!"

The doctor politely inquired, "Why don't you want to be examined?"

"I'm in terrible pain. After the examinations yesterday, I'm still suffering severe bleeding."

"Oh, in that case, go back to your room and rest. We're not going to bother you any more," he kindly assured me.

"Maybe you won't but others will."

"Nobody can do that to you if you're not feeling well."

That was encouraging, I trusted his words. I also knew it wasn't going to happen because I wouldn't permit it.

Two days after entering the hospital, the diagnosis confirmed my greatest fear.

I, Milenka Dobic, age 45, had Stage IV ovarian cancer, metastasized into my lymph system, liver and spleen. That was the hard hitting truth of the diagnosis on January 13th, 1987, but the doctors thought it best to conceal the truth from me.

Chapter 4

My Cancer is a Blessing

"Where is the left ovary? It looks like a huge cauliflower," a male pondered as he stared at the ultrasound monitor.

"Do you think we're going to get our raises at our next meeting?" a female wondered.

"Oh, for sure. Everybody is ready to fight for that. Look, I can't find the liver. This mess looks like thick fluid," another male opined.

"They have to do something because we haven't had any raises for the last six months. Do you want to know what I see there? Whole abdomen is one huge glob," a different female continued.

"We should speak to another division. If we stick together they'll have to give us our raises," chattered another unidentified individual.

Completely naked, with my bloated abdomen covered with oil, I lay on the table while their instrument glided over my body. I was listening to the borscht of their chatter. I was sure I must be hallucinating. None of this was real. I was invisible to them. To those six medical "experts" I was a lifeless cadaver.

"What about your Hippocratic oath? Where are your ethics?", I wanted to scream, "I'm a human being. You are describing my illness and I know what's going on. I have cancer!"

Without their invitation I sat up on the table.

"Will you tell me how sick I am?"

One female quickly answered, "Just wait a few more minutes and we'll be done."

"With what? Your raise or my case?"

A female jokingly responded, "With both, our raise and your case."

When they finished I asked the same question.

"Am I very sick?"

"Ask your doctor."

I got no answer from my doctor. A day after this examination my abdomen began to expand even more. Within 24 hours I looked nine months pregnant. Couldn't sit. Couldn't stand. The hundred pound "rock" I was carrying made my legs seem shorter. Couldn't sleep. I felt like I was choking. When I sat up in bed, my oxygen supply cut off. When I turned on my right side, my liver felt like it would explode. When I turned on my left side, numbness and pain forced me to try another position. Finally, I sat on the floor with my back resting against the bed. That enabled me to sleep but only for about half an hour.

"Oh, God, mercy. Please help me. What am I being punished for? Please don't let my children become orphans. Give me strength to endure this pain."

That night would have ended as a nightmare if I hadn't chosen to regale myself with all the happiest and funniest moments I had spent with my kids. Next morning God sent me Andrija. He found me in the hallway. While trying to conceal his anger his first question was, "Has the doctor seen you?"

"Yes. Yesterday morning but during the night I got worse. This morning I can hardly breathe." Saying that took my last breath.

"Let me find your doctor. I'll be right back."

Alone in the hallway, the thunder of my fear crushing me like 220 volts of electricity surging through my body. I knew what was coming. The usual prognosis of cancer was an early death! But then my natural spirit took over. I pictured Yelena, my six-year-old baby girl. I saw Srdjan, my fourteen-year-old son.

Then and there I made my commitment: I will survive. I will live. Instantly, my fear melted away. The thunder ceased. I was a fortress, impregnable, unyielding.

Andrija's voice sounded over my left shoulder.

"Mina, I think they're going to call you for surgery. I talked to the head surgeon. I told him that if they don't do something, I'm going to transfer you to my hospital. Did you eat anything this morning?"

"Andrija, how could I? I'm about to burst from holding all this fluid. There's no room for food. I lost my appetite two days ago."

When Bosko came for his usual visit he was wordless. The news of surgery sent shock waves through his heart. He began to perspire and paced anxiously. Color drained from his face. I saw his fear but he pooled all his reserves of strength to comfort me.

"Everything is going to be all right," he said. But his voice betrayed his real, deepest fears.

Andrija rested his arms on our shoulders in a reassuring gesture. "Everything is going to be O.K. Mina, be strong. See you after surgery." He looked away at nothing. The expression in his eyes belied his words. He left in a rush.

Smiling feebly, Bosko held me lovingly as we made our way back to my room. The nurse approached my bed and began preparing me for surgery. At 8 a.m. I was wheeled into the operating room. Bosko remained in the waiting room for the entire six hours of surgery.

As I was coming out of anaesthesia, I heard a man's voice whispering, "Too bad. There's no hope. She's such a young woman. Mina, Mina wake up."

I didn't want to wake up... ever. I was aimlessly drifting between consciousness and unconsciousness. My whole being gripped in the dark pangs of my abdomen, suffering without meaning. I forced my untamed subconscious to open my absent eyes, vacant of life. Strange feelings of emptiness and agony! My eyes touched the green, dreary walls of the operating room but it wasn't green enough.

I must leave! I must find a nicer green!

My imagination lifted me to a journey to the past; to the Green, Green Valley of my Birth Village. It is springtime. My unconscious is flooded with echoes of children's cheerful voices; whirling, tripping, dancing, as they eagerly chase after butterflies.

These delicate creatures spin around their heads, some landing on their hair, others fluttering up to sip nectar. I'm there! It's so vivid, so real, so warm. My body, drifting casually, again exists, senses, yet quivers all over with coldness.

A voice like piercing icicles says: *"Mina, Mina wake up, wake up."*

Where is that coldness coming from? It's real. It's chilling, painful. It's called reality. Let it go! Children's voices! Again I hear joyous screams, shrieks of laughter, sleds swishing over the snowy, silvery slopes — My White, White Valley. The overloaded sled plummets full speed down the hill, tumbling its cargo off. Noisy shouts of laughter, tangled bodies intertwined, wrestling, crawling, twisting together as they touch bottom. I must stay here and play. I must stay here till I die. Mirage! Familiar voices pull me out of this dream state.

"Srdjan, Yelena! Is that you?"

I opened my eyes wide, faintly amused. I felt remarkably well. Was that meditation?! (Meditation in my culture was virtually unheard of and at the least, frowned upon. I didn't realize it at the time but I had just discovered a new way of healing.)

This was a turning point in my recovery. It didn't matter what had happened those last six hours. I didn't have to know which part of my body was missing. What was important was feeling that nobody, nothing could separate me from my family, or take our love away.

I had discovered my purpose for living. I forgot the pain. An emotional dam broke through my chest larger and with more force than Niagara Falls. Now, as never before, I felt closer to my children and my beloved. I had almost lost them! I owed them my life, my soul. Each breath I breathed for them. This is my commitment! No tears, no sorrow.

Thank you, God. My cancer is a blessing for it taught me what is important in life.

The elevator doors slid open. Through a satiny mist I saw Bosko's face. He reached out and grasped my hand.

"Don't worry. Everything is going to be O.K. Now you're going to the recovery room," he whispered. He wanted to reassure me but I only heard his fear.

They wouldn't let him stay with me. As I lay there, fighting the sleep enveloping me, I heard a hushed voice, softly calling my name.

"Mina, Mina, Mina! Honey, don't be afraid. I'm with you!" It was Bosko! He had gotten as close to me as he could, positioning himself outside the recovery room near a small open louvre window. He was shivering in the minus 17 degrees Celsius that we call "Russian winter."

I knew it was Bosko, but I couldn't respond. My tongue was numb from anesthesia. In the same room, another woman had moaned and whimpered all night long. A sleepless night for me.

Then they moved me to intensive care with no visitors allowed. I couldn't see my husband for three days! Oh how I missed him! For the last twenty days, as faithfully as clockwork, Bosko had appeared at the foot of my bed each morning to comfort me. Those three days without him were eternity.

The doctors were amazed at how quickly I recovered. The day after surgery, I was able to refresh myself with a washcloth. The nurse was upset because she was supposed to do that for me. She didn't want me moving unnecessarily.

By the third day, I was well enough to return to the ward which I shared with four other women. All of us had cancer but we never talked about that. We were too busy having a good time, telling jokes, gossiping about everything and everyone, and teasing the doctors until they blushed. At times we were laughing so hard we were told to quiet down. We had a ball!

Bosko had had the answer to my question about cancer the day following the surgery. Early in the afternoon he had gone to my doctor's office.

"Don't worry. I fixed something. Everything is going to be O.K." the doctor reported proudly.

"Excuse me, doctor, are we talking about the same person?" Bosko inquired timidly, preparing to be disappointed.

The doctor was silent at first and then, "Oh, Oh... No, No, No." More restrained he asked, "How many children do you have, Bosko?"

"Two. A six-year-old daughter and fifteen-year-old son."

"I'm so sorry. Maybe she will live two months."

The reply was too emphatic for Bosko to doubt it. Contemplating the agony of his loss, he fainted. At the time, he didn't tell me what the doctor had said.

I had asked Bosko not to allow the children to visit me in the hospital. I didn't want them subjected to this stressful place. So you can imagine my surprise when I saw my son walking toward me. I jumped out of bed, spread my arms wide, raced toward him, hugging his trembling body as I guided him out of my room.

"You surprised me. I didn't know you were coming. Where's Daddy?"

"He's on a business trip."

Something in the way he said it caused me to doubt his words, although I had never known him to lie. Seeing him was just so unexpected, I wasn't sure what was going on. Only later did I find out the whole story. Bosko had been in bed three days with a high fever. He was gripped with fear, facing the cruel reality that he was losing me. That he and the children would have to live without me.

Holding tremulously to each other, Srdjan and I talked about everything.

"Daddy is behaving very strangely. I don't understand why he's so sad and depressed. Very often he leaves the room when we're watching TV. When I look for him, I find him crying. When I ask him why he's crying, he just says, 'Go back and watch TV.'"

"You know, for fourteen years, we've never been separated and it's hard for him. How are you? Do you miss me?" I asked Srdjan while kissing his forehead.

"Oh, yeah. I miss you a lot. I have you every night in my dreams. Like you're coming home passing through a valley full of colorful flowers. But I always wake up before you get home. Honestly Mommy, when are you coming home?" he pleaded.

I wished I knew the answer to that question. I couldn't get a straight answer from my doctor. Even the diagnosis wasn't clear to me. I didn't know what therapy they were going to recommend or how long it would take. But I answered him, "I promise, I will come home soon. Maybe only a few more...."

"What's a few?" he interrupted, tears smearing his pink cheeks.

"Days, my Sunshine — two, three days," I hugged him even tighter as he dived into my chest.

"Oh, Mother, I love you so much. I miss you terribly. Are you going to be O.K.?"

"I love you too. And I miss you more than anything. I'm O.K. believe me. I'm O.K. When I come home we will never be separated again. I'm going to get well and we're going to be happy. You just watch out for your little sister. Give her lots of love. And help Dad, don't ask so many questions. When I come home he's going to be different." We stood motionless, gripped in each others arms.

The head nurse approached, interrupting abruptly. In a totally detached voice and looking through me as if I were transparent, she inquired, "Are you Dobic?"

"Yes. I am Milenka Dobic."

"Get ready. We're moving you to another hospital. The car is waiting."

"How come? Which hospital? What for? Why didn't you tell me earlier? I want to talk to my doctor."

"O.K. Let me see what I can do."

Srdjan was noticeably agitated. "Mom, why do you have to go to another hospital?"

"Don't worry, Son. I'll keep my promise. I will not stay longer than two or three days. But I'm worried about how you'll get home. There's no direct bus line. And the bus station is far away."

It was so cold outside, mid-winter.

Again the nurse appeared, "Doctor wants to see you in his office right now."

"Wait for me here, Srdjan," I instructed. Hoping he couldn't hear the unevenness in my breathing.

I felt hacked and pulled. I moved slowly, taking deep breaths. I dragged myself with heavy steps to the doctor's office. Surgery had left me suffering with bleeding hemorrhoids, open, fiery, burning sores on my bottom. The doctor was friendly. He greeted me with kindness.

"Please be seated. What would you like to know?"

"Thank you. I prefer to stand. I want to know why I'm being moved to another hospital without explanation. I'm treated like a file, not a human being."

His face became flushed, "We're not equipped with proper facilities to treat your illness. The Oncology Institute in Sremska Kamenica has state of the art technology."

"Why do I need that special treatment? Is that chemotherapy?" I questioned, tensely expectant.

"You know we removed a tumor on the left ovary. We found damaged tissues in your abdominal area. There is also some dysfunction in your liver. But the major problem is that we couldn't remove the tumor, the size of a large grapefruit, that's still in your pelvic bone. That's what we have to treat with injections."

I interrupted him without taking a breath, "Do I have cancer? Is chemo what I'm going to get in that other hospital?"

"No. This is not chemo. And you don't have cancer," he insisted.

I moved impatiently, "But doctor, I feel I do have cancer and you don't want to tell me. I demand you tell me now. I'm a strong woman and I want to know my enemy so I know what I'm fighting. I'm not afraid because I know I'm not going to die."

Surprisingly, a smile flashed over his face, "I told you the truth, Mrs. Dobic. I'm glad to know you're such a strong woman. You'll need that in the future. But please get ready. My colleague from the Institute is waiting for you. We're sending your medical history with you for the oncologist at the Institute. Good luck, Mrs. Dobic."

Shaking his hand, I thanked him. I left his office and never looked back.

The nurse was waiting for me in front of the doctor's office and said she'd help me pack. We hurried because the chauffeur and doctor were waiting. We started to walk together in Srdjan's direction. With a disturbed tone in my voice, I told her, "I want my son to come with me."

"O.K. He can go. How old is your son?"

"Fifteen," I wasn't prepared for this conversation and so I may have responded coldly.

"Do you have more children?" she pushed the conversation further.

Her inquiry smacked of insincerity. She wasn't really interested in me personally. But rather, for reasons known only to her, she was on a fact-finding mission. "Yes, I have a six-year-old daughter."

As soon as we caught sight of Srdjan, our conversation ended.

They both helped collect my personal effects. On my way out to the car she hurriedly pushed two envelopes into my hands.

"Would you please give these to the oncologist. Good-bye." She whirled around and was gone.

I lost myself in a labyrinth of thoughts rendered unclear by my inability to reveal them. I still had so many unanswered questions floating around in my head. Secrets were being kept from me. So many half truths. No straight answers. It was a nightmare but only in bits and pieces, fragmented, disjointed and unconnected; tragic, yet provocative. Was it possible for someone to have cancer and not know it? And if that person did have cancer, why didn't the doctor just come out and say so?

But today something seemed different. For eighteen days I had lived without sunlight, fresh air and nature's holidays. Exultantly I walked out of that hospital with my precious son, hand in hand, greeted by the sun's tender waves of inconstant light warming my body. That marked a special moment in my life. For me it was the first day of the rest of my life. I was unstoppable! I had been released from prison… for a while.

Chapter 5

Choosing the Macrobiotic Way

The doctor was sitting in the front seat next to the chauffeur. I couldn't figure out what he was doing there. After all, how many people does it take to transport one small woman to a hospital? Later I got the answer. They gave me preferential treatment because they knew of my media affiliation.

Even more puzzling was why they gave me an unsealed envelope containing my diagnosis! They had gone to great lengths to conceal the truth from me. Would not logic dictate entrusting my records to the doctor travelling with us, rather than me?

So there I was. In the back seat of a luxury car, my son seated next to me, holding the unsealed secret report in my hands. I had a premonition of what was hidden inside that envelope. That's probably why I hadn't opened it immediately. If it was a secret to be hidden from the patient, why was it in the patient's hand? That strong doubt made me look inside.

Everything — the diagnosis, surgical procedure, after treatment, ongoing therapy — was all written in Latin. My knowledge of medical terms was limited but not my knowledge of Latin. I copied down the medical terms that I was unsure of. Later I would ask Andrija and Ratka.

I read it. My dreaded suspicions were confirmed. I had Stage IV terminal cancer, metastasized in my liver, my spleen and entire lymph system. The dismal truth filtered through. I glanced sideways. Srdjan was very quietly resting in the corner. He was yawning and rubbing his eyes. Tired from travelling 30 miles, riding two buses, walking to the hospital without having eaten lunch.

Half dazed I stuffed the papers back in the envelope. Idly gazing through the foggy window, I saw we were crossing a bridge over the icy Danube.

"Right here: it would be so easy to end my life. I have only to open the door and make my move. No, no, never!"

Angry at myself for such a thought. I wanted to scream, but not from sadness. It was more from the secrecy and deception that degraded me as a person. I had lost count of the times I had asked my doctor.

"Do I have cancer? Will I be treated with chemo?"

"No," had been his relentless reply.

He lied! But did he himself know why?

Srdjan sensed my fright. "Mom, what's happening? What are you thinking?" he murmured.

"I just don't want to leave you and go to another hospital."

"Why don't you come home with me?" his face lighting up with his well-thought-out solution.

"I have to sign some papers and go through some procedures before that can happen. We don't want the police to mistake us for escapees and chase us. But I promise you, in two days, I'll be home. There's nothing more they can do for me but there's plenty I can do for myself. And I think we should work on it together."

"Just tell me, Mommy, what I have to do," he offered proudly.

"When I return, we'll have a "Board of Directors" meeting. Our agenda will be: Number One — Srdjan will be the Disc Jockey charged with providing uninterrupted musical programs. Number Two — Daddy will be Chief Financial Officer in charge of bouncing checks. That'll keep him busy. Number Three — Yelena is Chief Assistant Cook to Mommy. That's a lot for a six-year-old but she can handle it. No, No, that's too easy. She'll have one more job. She'll also be in charge of entertainment. You know, stand around, smile broadly, laugh and giggle for no reason. At the same time, be Mom's official taster!"

Srdjan bent over, head bowed, holding his sides with peels of laughter, "Oh, this is great! What about you?"

"My job is to recover fast, so we can start living the happiest life ever. Have we got a deal?"

"We've got a deal, Mom."

"Oh, we're here already. Srdjan, don't you think it's best for you to go home and start working on this program right now? We all know you're good at that. And I'll get this hospital business out of the way, so I can be home soon."

"O.K. Mom," walking taller as he left.

Hugs, embraces and warm, sweet kisses were exchanged. I swelled with confidence at the thought of our short separation. Srdjan trotted off content, full of hope. As I walked toward the Institute I knew exactly how he felt, because I shared his feelings.

> *I go to my room. A sadness overtakes me. So I lie down on my bed, pull the covers over my head and instantly fall asleep. A reverie comes over me. Some kind of unknown courage is being born in me which is hidden and silent. In one moment of life's twilight, I feel a dull squeeze on my heart which is dark covered in blood every second. I see meninges beat ghastly, blind and hardly noticeable, barely shining ganglions, horrors of a body dying out. In the evening hour saturated with human closeness, I see unconsciousness and loneliness. A substance works and wears out cell by cell, dying out with no light and realization in a damned pain of fear; the kind of pain suffered by whatever lives, moves and dies. At this point I wish I were strolling along the beach, gazing upon sunsets, provoking platonic memories of the first tender love of my youth. I am desperately defending myself, calling up winds to blow away the cold in my veins so as to drive away the cramp in my body. I feel how each cell trembles and bristles in a duel. Then the sunset appears and consciousness wakes up to reign. In the bowels of my earth, when everything is ready to erupt, a volcano of self-confidence emerges, self-extinguishing before it actually hemorrhages. But that emotional doubting doesn't crush me with sorrow. I know the cancer can't kill the poet in me. My whole life is poetry from dawn to dawn. Every new dawning awakens in me a new greed for life.*

A moan awakens me. Reality impinges on my consciousness.

"I'm getting out of here!"

The next day, my new female doctor comes to my room to outline my treatment program. "Are you treating my cancer?" I want to know.

"Yes," her lips tightly compressed, her answer quick and sharp.

"Oh, thank you for telling me." Somebody finally told me the truth.

"Tomorrow morning we'll give you some papers to sign. That done, we can begin."

Arrangements were then concluded for chemotherapy and radiation. Of course, I had no idea how successful this treatment might be. I'd find out tomorrow and make my decision. That's why I felt no necessity to ask her any more questions.

I went to my room. These new hospital accommodations were much better than my previous ones. I stepped back and looked outside. The huge window opened onto a wondrous scene. Honey-colored sunlight silently announced its arrival, draping itself on the lip of a sleepy hollow. Majestic pine trees stood tall, commanding and feathery white, weighed down by glittering snow as it twinkled and fell to earth. My eyes were dazzled by stately mountains reaching heavenward, laced with soft cushions of snow, beckoning me to some secret hideaway.

That view was magical. For a brief moment I forgot the weariness of life. My lips parted in a delighted smile. My spirit lifted. It was a holiday for my eyes, fueling an insatiable thirst for life. Unreal — the frayed edges of my unconscious were jolted back to reality; a reminder of how far away we've strayed from appreciating nature's gifts. Oh, how talented an artist winter can be!

The other three women in my room were mired in suffering from the harsh, aggressive therapy. This excessive treatment caused an unnatural invasion of the senses which disconnected them from enjoying this glorious, exotic scene.

We were all cancer patients. The other women were already receiving chemotherapy and radiation. That was the rude reality. I was never able to really connect with my room-mates. Everyone was seriously ill. I was the healthiest of the "dying" cancer patients and I was ministering to their needs.

They were burning inside, asking me for lemon to moisten their dry, cracked lips. Their mouths were full of canker sores. Two of them had lost the use of their hands due to severe edema. One was totally bald. Her hair lost after the second, very aggressive chemo session. The oldest woman, 73 years, was babbling nonsense. They all looked medically abused.

"Is this going to happen to me? Is this the best I can expect? Is this therapy really healing or speeding up their demise?"

I recalled the words of Voltaire: "Doctors are men who prescribe medicines of which they know little, to cure diseases of which they know less, in human beings of which they know nothing."

I got my answer that night. The oldest roommate passed away. The doctor had no sooner left when I got a call from my doctor friend Ratka.

"How do you feel, Mina? Are you scared?" she asked casually.

"To be honest I feel pretty good. I'm not scared even after what I've just seen happen to the others. You know, Ratka, I'm ready to fight but not this way. I'm not going to take chemo or radiation."

Ratka's a no-nonsense, bottom-line kind of person. She asked bluntly, "You know you have terminal cancer. Did they tell you the prognosis if you're not treated with chemo and radiation?"

Ratka talked straight. She didn't mince words. "I talked to your doctor and she believes you have only two months to live."

This was the first time I had heard to prognosis. I exploded: "How can anyone know how terminal I am? If they already know the outcome, why are they recommending that treatment?!"

Somehow that news was a relief. It meant there was nothing more they could do for me.

"If that's true, then I'm going home." I certainly didn't want to spend the little time I had left rotting away inch by inch at the hands of a torturous therapy in this depressing environment.

"For heaven's sake, Mina, don't sign anything. I'm coming over right away."

Sure enough, she kept her promise. Ratka rushed into my room, sat down breathlessly and placed two books into my sweaty hands that ultimately shaped my destiny. One was entitled, *The Cancer Prevention Diet* by Michio Kushi and the other, *Recalled By Life,* by Dr. Anthony Sattilaro.

"Don't say "Yes" or "No", Mina, until you've read these books. Then you'll be better equipped to make your final decision."

The first book I read in four hours was Dr. Sattilaro's story. A magna cum laude graduate of Rutgers University, he completed medical studies at Hahnemann Medical College and Hartford Hospital. Became president of the Methodist Hospital in Philadelphia. He was diagnosed with terminal prostrate cancer, metastasized to his lungs and bones. Western medicine, of which he was a practitioner, gave up on him. He accepted macrobiotics as his approach and a year later was cancer free. If he can do it, I thought, so can I! I love this book. It is as simple as life itself.

Then I read two pages of *The Cancer Prevention Diet,* by Michio Kushi, translated into my language. They were about reproductive cancer. For the first time since my diagnosis I learned the true cause of my illness. Astonishingly, it was caused by an unbalanced diet!

Just looking at my half eaten lunch gave me a severe migraine. No more junk food for me! Back to the kitchen I sent the cheese, hot dogs, white bread and mocha coffee. "My God," I realized, "we're killing ourselves with food."

Better to fast at Lent than to put any more poison in my body. But what will I do about the nurses when I'm not eating. They'll never understand! So I devised a brilliant plan. I'll hide the plastic bags my sanitary napkins come in and conceal my food in them. Then nonchalantly saunter down the hall and quickly dump them in a trash can.

I was especially delighted to throw away the mucus forming cheese. I had learned it contributed to ovarian cancer. A long-remembered picture came to mind. It was Grandma. Her lifetime companion was an ashtray used as a spittoon. She used it to spit out gobs of heavy, yellow mucus coughed up from her lungs. Would you believe it? Her favorite food was dairy and especially my favorite, cheese. Kushi's book said that dairy, animal food, sugar and refined flour were the causes of ovarian and breast cancer. I had savored them all for 45 years! Of particular interest to us women is that this mucus concentrates in our female organs. Obviously the way to get well is to stop eating this food.

Just those few sentences turned my life around. I decided then and there, if there was any way to reach out for this strange and foreign alternative approach called macrobiotics, I'd do it. I wanted to. Yes, you see, it gave me hope! I had a short, sharp conversation with myself.

I said, "This is it! I'm going for it!"

It was nearly midnight when I called Ratka from the hall phone. She answered and heard the excitement in my voice. "I want to know what my chances are if I adopt the macrobiotic approach."

Her laughter resounded like a steeple bell. "I knew you'd like this and accept it. Mina, this is great. Leave the rest to me."

"I'm leaving for home tomorrow," my excitement still peaked. We were both talking at once.

"I'll be at your home tomorrow as soon as I finish work."

I floated two inches above the ground all the way back to my room. I had just won a fifty million dollar lottery! That night, I slept the sleep of the just.

Chapter 6

Home from the Hospital

It's five a.m. in the hospital bathroom. I'm already up using my make-up kit for the first time in twenty-two days. I'm talking to myself in the mirror.

"Today is your holiday. I'm going to make you pretty. An end to existing in darkness. I'll be with my children, my beloved, my friends."

I'm amazed. My body neither aches nor pains. I brush on some eye make-up. Nope, don't like that washed out green. Makes me look sick! I erase it. That soft mauve with a little brown looks much better. I look alive. I like the new me. I'm ready!

How do I get out of here without arousing suspicion? That'll take a little thought. Hmmm…. I got it! I'll spoof my doctor. Tell her I'm homesick, miss my family, dying to be home for the weekend. Promise her, "I'll be back Monday." Easy enough. She'll fall for that. Yes!

It's Friday, the 4th of February, 1987. One of the coldest, iciest winter days ever. Even the birds are hiding. Today I'll triumphantly close the hospital doors behind me. Rescued from my personal hell!

Bosko is still sick. He arranges for relatives to pick me up. The road is frozen. Dangerous. Like driving on a sheet of ice. The driver is inexperienced. Will he make it safely? Will my predicted two months be cut even shorter? Instead of forty-five minutes, it takes an hour-and-a-half to get home.

I'm prone on the back seat. The leather is hard and cold. Bosko's relatives are making conversation. They are trying to make me feel comfortable. But I can feel the chill of fear. I hear it and I see it. It's in their voices and their eyes. Sure that I'll die… they already feel sorry for me. I must escape from the cold. I crave the warmth of my loving family. My eyes close. I see them. Their dear faces surround me. My body yearns for the solace only they can give me. Even the seat beneath me is warmed. In my mind I'm home! I answer no more questions.

"She's sleeping," they say.

I'm warm and peaceful. After so much torture. Lies. Fake smiles. I'm going home.

The front door opens wide. My children rush to greet me — squealing, jumping, dancing, screaming, crying. They hug, squeeze and pet me. Oh how they love me! Dear Bosko still running a fever waits in line. He looks weak and drained. But seized with the exuberance and excitement of the homecoming, his fever takes flight.

Our friend Ratka Rudich, with her two babies, has moved in to care for me. She is busy in the kitchen, preparing my first macrobiotic meal. Miso soup, brown rice and steamed vegetables. "My savior," I cry as we hug each other.

What fun we had that weekend! Ratka scheduled my Saturday visitors at two-hour intervals between meal times. They had been instructed to leave their "sad face" at home. Relatives, friends and media colleagues brought entertainment with them. Harmonica, guitar, violin, joined in a chorus of voices filling our home. I joined them. Jokes and laughter echoed through the open windows. Passers by remarked, "The Dobics are having a party." The celebration lasted into the night. Forty people came and went that day. This is the way to get well!

Everybody wanted to taste my "new" food. They all said, "I love it." The conversation took a deeper philosophical turn. When humankind ate naturally, we were healthier. Less meat, less sugar, no processed foods. There was little illness. I knew my friends were being kindly supportive. The truth is, despite their compliments, I knew it would be difficult for them to change their way of eating, way of life. I had an advantage. Cancer threatened my life. I was motivated. I wanted to live. That meant no eating out.

I had bleeding hemorrhoids. Hospital medications had caused inflammation in the genital area. I was forced to use cotton gauze and sanitary pads for the bleeding. One weekend changed all that. Amazing grace! Simple macrobiotic meals for two days. The bleeding stopped. My hemorrhoids healed. "Yes, Hippocrates, food is our best medicine."

Bosko had his first lesson in macrobiotics. He barely tasted some of my food. We both knew I was going to get well. Yelena and Srdjan loved my brown rice with gomashio. (See Glossary) That weekend altered the life of my whole family.

Monday morning Bosko and I returned to the hospital. We stayed just long enough to inform my oncologist Maria Teshic, Ph.D., that I had decided to pursue an alternative approach. She appeared to be shocked. Her mouth opened but uttered no sounds. Then briefly tripping over her words, she regained her composure, "Well, you can't do that. If you leave, you cannot come back any more."

Now it was my turn to be shocked. With appropriate indignation, I asked expansively, "Why not? Whose policy is that? Who passed that law? I have been contributing to my own health care program for thirty-six years. I've paid for health care. I have the right to it and I'll be back as the need arises."

Leaning forward, eyes riveted to mine, afraid to offend, Dr. Teshic asked softly, "What is the name of your new approach?"

"Macrobiotics," I said full of assurance, not hesitating at all. That word filled the room. Hearing the commitment in my voice, she sensed I couldn't be dissuaded. To our surprise, she told us she was familiar with macrobiotics.

"Neither my family nor I eat meat," she confided. "We eat soya products, brown rice, beans and fish."

All her colleagues ate meat for breakfast, lunch and dinner. How could she possibly share with them how good she felt eating macrobiotically? They would consider the whole idea absurd. She protectively suggested that any time I wanted tests she would arrange for them and expedite the results. She wanted to stay in touch. That was the first support I had from practitioners of Western medicine. Renewed and refreshed, we left.

I was relieved but Bosko wasn't. The far off look in his eyes betrayed his fear that in two months he would lose me. Nevertheless on our way home we sang and talked about the plan for our new way of life.

Home again. My regime changed 360 degrees. Ratka carefully arranged my daily schedule. I followed it blindly, willingly. My family didn't understand either but no one objected.

Morning started at 5 a.m. in the bathroom. Bosko vigorously scrubbed my body with a hot ginger water towel until my whole body tingled and became red. Then Bosko left for work.

I went downstairs to the living room and exercised: yoga stretches; self-massage by pounding each meridian with my fists from head to toe; bringing energy to the surface.

Next, to the kitchen for breakfast. Seated around the table were myself, my daughter, Ratka and her eldest daughter. It was chew, chew, chew and think positive thoughts. Every bite 200 times. Ratka brooked no disturbance. No talking, no phone, no interruptions. It was a quiet breakfast as you can imagine. Broken only by the sounds of determined chewing. It lasted from 8:00 to 8:50 a.m.

She instructed, "Chewing each bite 200 hundred times causes your saliva to produce digestive enzymes, and nutrients enter the blood stream more speedily to nourish the cells and strengthen your immune system." True. And the more I chewed, the better the food tasted. Ratka was the only doctor I knew that made the connection between food and health.

I loved my cup of miso soup which Ratka made with wakame seaweed, vegetables and barley miso. The label on the miso container read: "Prepared with deep well water, barley and soya beans — both certified organic — unrefined sea salt and koji culture-starter. Aged in wooden vats for a minimum of three summers, no preservatives or additives." It sounded very Japanese!

"Where do you get all the ingredients," I asked her.

"From abroad. Nothing is available locally. Everything has to be imported."

My "medicine" made me feel good. We had lots of soft short grain brown rice with kombu seaweed and well water; steamed vegetables — more cabbage and carrot tops than root vegetables. We didn't have enough macrobiotically cooked food for everyone, so my family ate with me only twice a day.

After lunch, I took a half-hour walk. Weather permitting, Yelena went with me. Each day my walk exhausted me more. Ratka explained that my body was detoxifying. The enzymes that dissolve fat and mucus are created by exercise. After dinner I took another half-hour walk, this time with Bosko. We carried a small stool on which I sat for rest as needed. I was concerned about the weakness in my legs, so heavy and slow moving.

Again Ratka patiently explained, "You stuffed your body with fatty foods for many years and now it's eliminating all those toxins, fat and mucus which your body has been holding."

"O.K. If you say so. You're my doctor — my guardian angel," was my trusting answer.

For me there was no longer any rushing, running, stressing myself. I welcomed this regime and embraced it with ease. I knew I could maintain it after Ratka left. In the very first week, a sense of calm and peace overtook me. Even the children sensed it and played together without fighting and screaming. No loud voices were heard in our home. Where was this change coming from? Could the food be doing this? Does that mean food is energy? If food is energy, why was I still so weak?

Ratka gave me the answer. "Meridians and channels within the body correspond to each organ. If there is stagnation or excess, the body reacts with discomfort or pain. If the condition becomes chronic, tumors, cancer or other illnesses result. Pain is the body's signal that it's getting rid of something harmful. If we exercise vigorously, it speeds the body's process of detoxification. At first, this makes elimination more extreme. That's the reason for your weak legs."

Ratka had been with us four weeks. She stayed another week to organize our trip to the Kushi Institute, in Boston, U.S.A. Responding to her solicitations, relatives, co-workers, and close friends donated money for our trip. In a week-and-a-half, everything was arranged, including two round trip tickets from Belgrade to Boston.

Bosko was going with me. The children were to stay with relatives. Ratka gathered all the information we needed about The kushi Institute and Michio Kushi.

Chapter 7

First Trip to U.S.
A Celebration of Life!

I began 1987 renewed. I had cancer in my body but hope in my heart. I was going to live! My children would not be orphans. I knew my enemy. Ignorance led to cancer, but enlightenment heals. I was going to fight. I joined nature, and nature always wins.

One glorious Monday my media friends came to our home, waving our tickets over their heads. Altogether they had donated $8,000. They brought music, singing and dancing with them; their light-hearted spirits infected us all. Everyone swayed to the rhythm of rejoicing. Our home was blessed with unconditional love. On Friday we'd be on our way to the United States!

Bosko and I were having mixed feelings, different feelings. It wasn't fear of our expected trip because that was to be a journey of healing. It must have been the stress of the change. It felt like a tickling in my chest. I noticed the wrinkles on Bosko's forehead had deepened and tightened. Perhaps it was just the need to divest ourselves of our old habits; of thinking we had to run our own lives instead of trusting the matchless creative powers of the universe.

Our children were excited and happy. Mom and Dad were going to America. They'd be bringing goodies from "wonderland." We were going first to New York City. Mladja, one of Bosko's New York business associates, gladly accepted the invitation to be our host. He agreed to serve as our contact person and guide. His office was located in the Empire State Building, in the capital city of the world!

Packing was the easiest part of the trip. Mladja advised us to pack plenty of warm clothing as extremely cold winters are the rule rather than the exception. We had one large piece of luggage between us for our clothes and two extra-large suitcases for diapers. No, we weren't importing them, nor expecting a baby. Surgery had left me with a steady, watery vaginal discharge.

I used thirty or more diapers every twenty-four hours. Since factories in our country had long since ceased producing them, Bosko had had to travel to Austria to get them. During the cold winter months, it was especially burdensome. When I got wet I felt even colder. I had to change diapers more often.

Thursday night, our phone rang nonstop for six hours. Everyone wanted to say good-bye. That was an especially delightful experience as the entire event was broadcast on Radio Indjija. Good wishes poured in all night long: "We are with you. We want to see you back, happy, strong, on your way to full recovery."

Friday morning at 8 o'clock our front yard became a huge parking lot. There were enough bouquets to start our own flower shop. My eyes glanced to and fro among the crowd, searching for faces of relatives and friends. Our house was wall-to-wall with people coming to say their farewells.

In our country an event of this magnitude was usually a wedding or some other traditionally happy occasion. This was not traditional, it was exceptional. The heavens had opened up and showered upon me a blessing I could not have imagined. This mountain of support reaffirmed my belief that I was going to win this fight. The only one crying was Bosko's mother. The children were trying to console her.

"Grandma, don't worry. Mom and Dad are coming back next week and they're going to bring us presents from America. If you cry you won't get any," my round, egg-shaped six-year-old baby girl cautioned her.

A large group of relatives and friends remained at our house to comfort those staying behind, waving until we were out of sight. But an even larger convoy of vehicles trailed behind our car all the way to the airport. An undeniable feeling of exhilaration surged through my frail body. If only I had wings, I could fly to America just on my own power! Friends from the radio station shared our car. Someone turned on the radio and I heard my favorite song. Then the D. J. announced: "To our dear Mina: All the listeners of Radio Indjija are wishing her a safe trip and happy return with medicine for her long life."

We never stopped singing. If we'd had a car phone we could have called that D.J. and asked to have our singing recorded live on radio. Usually it takes nearly an hour to get to the airport. We made it in much less time. At least it seemed that way. The traffic lights were all green. I think it was prearranged!

I was confident and self-assured, talking arrogantly to the cancer: "Now what do you think? Who is going to win? You'd better give up right now. You don't have a chance. You have no friends, no relatives and I bet you my healthy cells are tripling by the second. Aren't you jealous? You'd better be. You don't have much more time. Prepare to be terminated!"

At the airport, more family and friends were waiting: my father, my brother, my sister-in-law. The exhilarating sendoff made my trip a celebration of life, a treasure chest of love. After an endless number of warm hugs and kisses, Bosko and I boarded the plane. As our flight began, I started re-reading *The Cancer Prevention Diet* by Michio Kushi but this time with more understanding and appreciation. The unnatural, artificial environment of the plane challenged my body's resources. Every half hour I found myself making a trip to the restroom.

Ratka had prepared a delicious macrobiotic meal for me to take on the flight. When meal time came I devoured my sushi with rice, vegetables and seaweed, followed with a cup of warm bancha tea. I was content. Even more so when Bosko asked to share my food. That was a first for him. We both knew the worst food on planet earth is served on aeroplanes and cruise ships. I survived those twelve hours with good food and emptied one suitcase of diapers.

Twenty-four hours later we arrived at John F. Kennedy Airport in New York. Our contact, Mladja, was supposed to be waiting for us. But that wasn't the case. It was February 17th, President's Day and everything was closed, even Mladja's office. Bosko tried to reach him but was unsuccessful.

Bosko spoke English very well but I didn't. Ratka had written down the address and phone number of The kushi Institute. Outside the airport we handed the paper to a cab driver. He looked at the address and 617 area code. Then looked at us with an, "Are you kidding me?" look.

"I have to call this number here in Brookline," Bosko said expectantly.

Laughing sourly the cab driver muttered, "Brookline? No sir, this ain't Brookline. This here's Brooklyn, New York. Brookline's about five hundred miles northeast of here in Boston, Massachusetts."

Bosko nearly fainted on the spot. Tiny droplets of perspiration appeared on his forehead betraying his fear. Poor Bosko. But that was only the beginning of this adventure.

"Are you sure about that?" Bosko begged, forgetting his timidity.

"I'm positive! You can get there by plane, bus or train." The cabby licked his lips and spoke in a half jeer.

After the initial shock Bosko and I had a quick conference. He decided to call Ratka and asked the cab driver to wait.

"O.K. I'll wait, but it'll cost ya'," nodding gravely.

Bosko was one step away from terrified — a sick wife, limited finances. Despite his trembling hands, Bosko finally reached Ratka. She consoled him with a logical comment, "Bosko, five hundred miles north, south, doesn't matter. You're still in the United States."

Our view of the U.S. was tainted by Hollywood and especially the movie "Cab Driver." In all the movies we had seen the bad guys were always black… and mean. This cab driver just happened to be black. His compact, sinewy body, towering persona and loftiness were evenly matched. As I look back, I can hardly forgive myself for such a distorted misconception. In our case it wasn't racism. It was just plain ignorance.

We decided to find a modestly priced hotel close to Mladja's office and call him in the morning. Somehow we herded ourselves into the cab. Not more than five minutes later, Bosko glanced up just in time to catch the cabby looking at him in the rear view mirror. With one hand on the wheel and the other holding a phone, we heard the cabby, with a blood-curdling snarl, warn:

"One more word and I'll kill you."

Bosko looked over at me. I looked back at Bosko. Is this a movie? Oh, my God. Did we come 5,000 miles to die at the hands of a murderous lunatic? Shocked into silence my dear husband reacted to what he perceived to be an impossibly dangerous situation. His body began a full range of involuntary contortions; his whole body shrank deeper into the seat. His left hand started to twitch ever so slightly. His eyes widened, then gloomily squinted almost shut. He blushed like a school boy after his first kiss.

Bosko bent over, bowed low, resting his elbows on his knees and holding his head in his hands. Then quickly, shifted his right hand over his stomach, caressing it ever so gently. His chalky lips dropped open. A faint, ghostly moan ran over his lips. In the dim shadow, I saw just a hint of saliva collecting in one corner of his mouth. I was about to ask him if he was all right. Just in time, Bosko collected himself and somehow got the words out, breathless but politely:

"Sir, I'm not feeling well. Would you please pull over?"

Bosko discharged all his stress, including everything he had eaten the last twenty-four hours, in a parking lot somewhere on the outskirts of New York! Poor Bosko, that was an embarrassing scene for him. But I knew the goal of our journey and I didn't care what the driver of the cab might think.

Thus on President's Day we arrived in front of the President's Hotel, two blocks from the Empire State Building. From our initial despair our perspective of black people changed dramatically due to the kindness of our cab driver. He helped us to the reservations desk, took our suitcases upstairs and refused to take more than $30 for everything. He made us feel welcome in a strange and unfriendly city.

"God Bless you sir and ma'am. Good luck," were his final words as he politely waved good-bye.

This city greeted us with frantic chaos and noise reserved for such notable criminals as Al Capone! Blaring police sirens, screeching ambulance sirens, fire engine sirens blasting in concert.

"Is it always like this? What's going on here?" I couldn't help asking myself. This is a strange place. In our country, if we hear a siren once in six months, that's a lot. We found out later, there'd been a robbery at a nearby bank.

Our hotel accommodations were quite satisfactory. I was excited. I wanted to take a walk around Manhattan. I was dying to see Broadway but Bosko didn't want to go anywhere. It was only 5:30 p.m. when he went to sleep. I managed to have fun by myself. I watched the activity at a valet parking lot below our window. Limousines (we don't have these at home) were coming and going, dropping off casually dressed guests at a restaurant.

I wanted to take a short walk to see the front of that restaurant. But, not speaking the language, I didn't dare venture out on my own. The longer I stood at the window and smelled those tantalizing Italian aromas, the hungrier I became. I decided to have supper by myself. What a terrible disappointment. All the food Ratka prepared had spoiled. There was nothing left to eat. I didn't have the courage to wake Bosko and try to locate a macrobiotic restaurant. I knew he wouldn't go. I tried once more to reach Mladja, without success.

That evening I worked very hard on my mind and consciousness. I did visualization. Welcomed our kids into our room, followed by yoga. Around 8 o'clock I fell asleep. The next morning I was awakened by Bosko's voice.

"Great, Mladja, we'll be ready in half-an-hour. Thank God we found you."

"Don't worry, I'll arrange everything," he assured us.

We weren't sure if the money we had would cover all our expenses. After talking with Mladja, we decided to travel to Boston by Greyhound to conserve funds. Unfortunately, we got seats positioned directly over the wheels in a bus that had no shock absorbers! By the end of that five-and-a-half-hour ordeal, every inch of my body cried out in pain. And I had already spent twenty-four hours without nourishment. I refused to eat any food that was not macrobiotic and we hadn't had time to find a macrobiotic restaurant. We arrived in Boston at 1 a.m.

We had come all this way without an appointment with Michio Kushi, not knowing whether he was even in the country. Fortunately, Attea, a lovely Greek girl who was the secretary in charge of scheduling his appointments, was able to book a consultation. It was at 5 p.m. on the 22nd of February, 1987, the day before he was leaving for Japan. Such good fortune could only have been God's will.

We fell in love with Boston and instantly felt at home. It reminded us of Europe. People looked less lost. We stayed at the Anthony Townhouse at 10850 Beacon Street, furnished in early American. It was clean, warm, friendly and safe. Our hostess, Barbara, greeted us with a broad, warm smile. I forgot about food. I slept until 10 a.m. — my third day without food. Attea, a Greek angel, arranged lunch for us at the Kushi Institute.

To get there, we had to take the inbound subway. It was a 15 minute walk on one of the coldest, windiest days of that winter. My feet were heavier than iron, my rusty knees were creaking with frostbite. I had lost so much weight, my slacks had to be pulled up, folded over and crudely knotted so I wouldn't lose them in an embarrassing moment. Finally we arrived in front of the Kushi Institute at 17 Station Street in Brookline, Massachusetts. Two more flights of stairs to go. I prayed this ascent meant getting closer to good health.

I loved the Kushi Institute. I loved the smell of the food. Everything was clean and holy. I couldn't hold back the tears, I hugged Bosko. "Honey, we're here. I'm going to live. I just know it."

They prepared a macrobiotic feast for us. With eyes closed, I chewed my warm miso soup, saying a prayer of thanks with each mouthful. Rice, steamed vegetables with kabocha squash, arame seaweed dish, black soybean stew and pressed salad. Bosko had two extra croquettes. We savored every mouthful. That was a delightful day!

Then we met a couple from Yugoslavia who were studying at the Institute. Dragomir and Seka Vukovich were lovely, friendly people. They helped us immensely. We had dinner together at Open Sesame Restaurant. We were in Shangri-La. Food was luscious. We had new friends, an appointment with Mr. Kushi. We celebrated life with lots of laughing, singing, joking and dancing. I'll treasure those days until the end of my life. Next day, we were scheduled to begin the three-day Way of Life Seminar. We had enough money to buy needed food. No question about it, God wanted me to live. We lacked nothing.

From the first bite of the Nishime dish at the Open Sesame Restaurant, I felt fulfilled. I chewed and I chewed and I chewed. The meal was well balanced. The food full-flavored and delectable. I was seated opposite Bosko. He leaned toward me, wiping my tears away with his handkerchief.

"Honey, it's O.K. We're here. Don't worry." He touched my cheeks with so much love. I'm sure everyone in the restaurant felt those loving vibrations, too.

"I'm not crying because I'm sad. I'm crying because I'm happy. I'm so grateful that I'm here. I want to hug all these people. And I adore you for everything that you've done for me. Thank you, my love."

Then I thanked our waitress for serving us and asked her to thank the cooks for the delicious meal. I invited her to choose something from the menu as our gift. She humbly accepted a small glass of carrot juice.

I sensed a difference in the atmosphere of that restaurant. The view wasn't anything special. Just houses with snow-topped roofs and a parking lot. Decor was simple but to me everything was perfect. Patrons were quiet. Staff were smiling and friendly. A genuinely warm, caring, calm atmosphere pervaded the room. I remember how cold I was before I walked in and how warm I was when I left. We didn't take the subway back to the Inn. We walked. We sang. We danced in the street.

We arrived at our room in no time. Bosko and I nearly squeezed the life out of poor Barbara who happened to be in the hallway. She couldn't believe that we were the same two people who registered the day before. An amazing transformation had taken place right before her eyes.

"What's happened?" she asked.

Bosko answered, "We found a treasure and we are rich."

"Where? Tell me, I'd like to be rich too. You've just arrived and you're rich already?"

Bosko told her the thrilling story of our discoveries, event by event. Meeting all those friendly people at the Kushi Institute, Open Sesame Restaurant and the delicious meals at both places; our good fortune to have scheduled an appointment with Mr. Kushi just two days from now; our new-found friends from Yugoslavia who were going to act as interpreters; how everything was falling into place for us. I wished I could have spoken English. I would have told her myself. But I did exactly that a few years later after I learned the language.

Moreover, after just one day of being in a healthy environment and being on a macrobiotic diet for almost two weeks, I felt like a billion dollars. I believe that my body started healing at that moment. Is that possible? Is that a miracle? Well, I believe in miracles.

Seeing cooking classes on the Institute schedule made me worry less. This meant I'd know how to prepare my own food once I got home. That evening I was too excited to sleep. I was up early scrubbing my body with a hot towel, without Bosko's help — almost singing. I say "almost" because people were still sleeping and I didn't want to disturb them. My chest was too small for the emotions I was holding. My spirit was ready to take flight. Fear was gone. Faith took over. In an instant I felt the whole world supporting me. And love, the only energy in the universe, filled the chapel of my soul, my skinny petite body. I was wealthy. I didn't need anything else. Love was enough.

The next day, Bosko and I were the first to arrive at the Kushi Institute. We were standing in front of the classroom door, excited in expectation of all the new knowledge we were about to receive. The class was full. There were people of all ages and more than fifty percent of them had cancer.

"Introduction to Macrobiotics," the first lecture, was taught by Edward Esko, a very powerful and dynamic educator. We were seated in the back row. As he spoke, my new friend Seka leaned over and whispered in my ear, translating each word. I was paying more than the usual attention to everything she said. I couldn't believe what I heard, the simplicity of it. The logic of living life in a natural way, in harmony with nature.

The message was: by eating in harmony with nature and your environment you will create order and balance in your daily life. You don't have to change your religion. Being harmonious will shift your way of thinking and way of life. (See Appendix A for more details about macrobiotic philosophy.)

We also learned that the macrobiotic diet is based upon native common sense and intuitive understanding of the relationship between humanity and the environment. A peaceful spirit will extend to family, community and eventually influence the whole world. In the Western world meat; poultry and eggs; milk, cheese and other dairy foods are the backbone of the modern diet. Physiologically, they give the human organism an immediate burst of energy and strength. But a heavy, meat-centered diet can have adverse effects on human health. Meat starts decomposing as soon as an animal is killed. It is harder to digest than plant foods and continues to putrefy in the digestive tract, taking about four hours to be absorbed in the intestines as compared with only two hours for grains and vegetables. Putrefaction produces toxins that accumulate in the liver, kidneys, and large intestine, destroys bacterial culture and causes degeneration of the villi of the small intestine where metabolized food is absorbed into the blood. Saturated fat raises the amount of cholesterol in the blood. Saturated fatty acids, from meat and other animal products, accumulate in and around vital organs and blood vessels, often leading to cysts, tumors, and hardening of the arteries.

"Scary and so overwhelming. Why didn't they teach us this in school? Why did we choose poison instead of food?" was Bosko's question.

During the break and snack, we got to meet and talk to others. Six of them had already recovered from cancer. They were optimistic and willingly shared their experiences. That gave us more confidence and hope. Bosko and I agreed that this was the best investment we'd ever made in our entire life.

Ahhh — what a snack! They served delicious cornbread with roasted tahini, miso and squash spread and bancha tea. From the very first bite of the cornbread, with its sweetness caressing my taste buds, it was deja vu. I was reliving this experience knowing I had done this at an earlier time. Where and when, I didn't know.

During the break one woman wasn't feeling well. She had digestive problems and cramps, and had to lie down. A couple of minutes later one of the staff brought her a special medicinal drink with a very strange name: Ume-Sho-Kuzu. Shortly after taking the drink she felt much better. We all wondered what was in it. The girl who brought it told us *umeboshi* is a special kind of plum, pickled for nine years in sea salt with Japanese leaves called *shiso*. Also in the drink were *kuzu*, a white, sticky powder and *soy sauce*. It didn't matter to me what they called it. It only mattered that it worked!

After the break, we agreed that people in our Yugoslav homeland used to live very close to the macrobiotic way. That's the way we had been raised. I jumped into the middle of the conversation.

"I remember when I was young, we only ate meat three times a month. Our whole family had twenty-five pounds of sugar for the entire year! On special occasions we had cookies. Adults got one, kids got two. Other kinds of desserts were reserved for guests. I don't remember getting sick more than once or twice a year.

"When we were poor, we couldn't afford meat or sugar. When we got more money, we started eating meat and sugar every day. We got sick more often, too. Many still suffer from high blood pressure, migraines, lower back pain, arthritis, and God knows what else."

At that point, the lecture resumed. The atmosphere warmed. It was like old friends getting together for a special occasion.

The speaker presented new ideas: "To compensate for eating meat, poultry, eggs, and other animal foods, the body requires more oxygen in the bloodstream. The breathing rate rises after eating animal food, making it difficult to maintain a calm mind. Thinking in general becomes defensive, suspicious, rigid, and sometimes aggressive. A very narrow, analytical view is often the result.

"Dairy food affects all organs and systems. Because it is a product of the mammary gland, it primarily affects the human glands, especially the reproductive organs. The most commonly affected are the breast, uterus, ovaries, prostate, thyroid, nasal cavities, pituitary gland, the cochlea in the ear, and the cerebral area surrounding the midbrain. It appears first as the accumulation of mucus and fat, then the formation of cysts, tumors, and finally cancer. Dairy also produces mucus accumulations resulting in hay fever and hearing difficulty. Other common problems include vaginal discharges, ovarian cysts, fibrosis and uterine cancer, ovarian cancer, and prostate tumors."

"He's talking about my case," I whispered in Seka's ear.

"Mina, you are right on!" Seka complemented.

"This extreme way of eating causes contraction in the organs and the body craves expansive energy to balance — creating yet another extreme — mankind's foremost poison: sugar. Excessive sugar suppresses the immune system, inhibits liver function, and causes energy loss, depression and obesity. Simple sugar lacks vitamins, minerals and fiber, and depletes the body of its own store of minerals and co-enzymes for metabolization. Sugar literally burns the body's nutrients and causes acidity. Could that be why the most reported symptom in this country is 'lack of energy'?

"White sugar uses up Vitamin B, without which the body is unable to utilize glucose. The brain and eyes only use glucose, a sugar, for fuel. When glucose levels are low the brain does not receive enough energy to function properly. According to researchers at Georgetown University, Washington, DC, twenty million Americans suffer from carbohydrate sensitivity and sugar is a pure carbohydrate! Daily use of sugar causes the pancreas to produce more insulin and leads to chronic hypoglycemia and diabetes.

"Sugar turns into fat. Fluctuations of blood sugar cause a number of other side effects: anxiety, irritability, headaches, uncontrolled emotions, poor memory and poor concentration. It also has been linked to confusion, dizziness, hyperactivity in children, nightmares, increased aggressiveness, anti-social behavior, suicidal tendencies and mental illness.

"Sugar is a major contributor to intestinal cancer, peptic ulcers, appendicitis, inflammation of the gall bladder and hemorrhoids."

From what I learned that day, I made a very simple chart:

> Sugar affects nervous system,
> → adversely affects the brain,
> → leading to depression,
> → psychiatrist.
> Solution: treat the cause — stop consuming simple sugar!

For the first time in my life, I learned that one of the causes of common illnesses in the worldwide population is excessive intake of saturated fats and cholesterol. The arteries become clogged, eventually leading to strokes and coronary problems. Animal fats collect toxins from the animal's body. We assimilate these toxins when we eat their fat.

Bosko and I couldn't believe our ears! Our favorite foods were poison!

The speaker continued: "One egg, one chicken. Eggs have an 'ascending direction,' which influences energy and fluids to move higher in the body. Traditional Chinese medicine claims eggs contribute to liver related conditions such as vertigo, strokes, nervousness, spasms, and paralysis. Eggs create an extremely sticky mucus forming quality which can eventually obstruct the gall bladder, slow the functioning of the liver, and leave deposits throughout the body."

The macrobiotic diet was introduced at that three-day seminar as the most balanced diet. We had already sensed that. I cannot tell you in detail what else we heard. Later we got more information from literature about food and its energy. Otherwise, we would have been too confused and lost in our new dietary understandings.

We learned so much about life, about our relationship with the universe, Earth, and our bond with Nature. We learned more about life in those three days than in all our past forty years. We had no doubts. We had no questions. We understood the simplicity of nature's law, the natural way of living. Jokingly on our way home, we said that Columbus discovered America but we discovered the facts of life by coming here. And it didn't take us nearly as long to discover the real life as it took him to discover America!

The most exciting part of this life-giving education was the cooking class conducted by Mary Kat, a very strong Irish woman and macrobiotic teacher. We learned how to make miso soup, pressure-cooked rice, azuki beans with squash, pressed salad and kanten for dessert. We learned that macrobiotic food is medicine. Each dish has a specific medicinal purpose.

The general nutritional guidelines given were: use more basic carbohydrates, fewer simple carbohydrates; more good quality vegetable protein rather than animal food protein; drastically reduce fat and use more unsaturated or less saturated fat. Also, we learned about the need to balance various natural occurring vitamins, minerals and other nutritional factors. And to use more organically grown, natural quality food, unprocessed and free of chemicals. Emphasis was placed on consuming whole foods as opposed to refined and partial foods.

We understood that our future food was going to consist mainly of whole grains, beans, soy products, sea vegetables, pickles, seeds, condiments, and occasionally fish and fruit. To be able to cure cancer and sustain the immune system, the foods that must be avoided were those we had been eating all our life.

When the cooking class was over we got to sample the recipes. Each dish had its own unique flavor. In one meal we had salty, sour, pungent, bitter, and sweet; composed with balance that satisfied our palate. The presentation of the food, the various colors on the plate, were visually pleasing. It was beyond food. It was art.

We were overjoyed to learn food could prevent illness; as well as heal illness. The first day I asked myself: how am I going to manage this when I get home. Very little was known about macrobiotics in my country. I was in the media for eleven years and had never heard the word "macrobiotic." There was no macrobiotic center in my country. There was no one there to answer my questions when I asked them. Nor was there any one who would be able to help me, or guide me through my recovery. But none of this discouraged or frightened me. I'm a visual learner and I watched the teacher closely.

As soon as the class was over, Bosko and I ran to the health food store a few doors away and bought a pressure cooker, miso paste, short grain brown rice, dry shiitake mushrooms, kombu and wakame seaweed. Having these basic ingredients made me calm and confident. I knew I could do it.

One day remained of the seminar before my appointment with Michio Kushi. After merely five days we had already noticed physical and emotional changes. Fear seemed to fade away, calm reigned supreme. No arguments, no loud voices speaking disagreeable words. Our doubts took wing. We sensed a closeness and oneness which connected us in a more deeply rooted love and happiness which persists to this very day. That is our shared miracle!

Chapter 8
Michio Kushi

February 22nd 1987, we had our scheduled consultation with Michio Kushi. He is the founder of the East-West Foundation and the acknowledged leader of the international macrobiotic community and natural food movement. A renowned healer, he teaches people how to overcome their illness with a special dietary approach and lifestyle change.

I met him first through macrobiotic books. Some of our friends thought of him as "that strange Japanese man who thinks food can cure cancer." But everything he said made sense to me. It was logical and clear — to live in harmony with nature's law. I lived that way as a child but had forgotten this wisdom.

On our way to the consultation, we guessed how Mr. Kushi would look. Bosko was sure of his vision. "You will see. He is a little shorter than me, round face, and small eyes like a fish, just like all Japanese people. His hair is black and perfectly combed. He will be dressed professionally, wearing a suit and tie."

My guess was not too different. Except I guessed he was taller, had a high forehead and was slender and elegant.

Seka and Dragomir were waiting for us in the lobby of the Institute. Dragomir told me he was going to transcribe as well as translate for us. That was a provision from God. After fifteen minutes, the receptionist advised us that Michio Kushi would see us. When we walked into the room, it reminded me of a classroom. Mr. Kushi was there, alone, a refined gentleman, slim, tall, dressed in a smart dark blue suit. The color suited him well. His warm smile welcomed us as he reached out to shake our hands. He didn't look anything like we had imagined.

I'll always remember the way his spirituality dominated his physical form. He radiated a calmness and his peaceful spirit filled the room. His gracious manner immediately put us at ease and satisfied our need for contentment and peace. Instinctively we knew he possessed extraordinary healing power.

Suddenly every cell in my body felt energized. This humble and mild-spirited man had already dispelled all doubts and fear. In one fleeting moment, I believed his assurance that my hope was well placed.

Looking directly into my eyes, he said simply, "In one year you can get well if you do what you learn here." Then he turned to Bosko and said, with an equal amount of conviction, "Yugoslav people have very strong constitutions."

That was his first verbal contact with us. Bosko, under the influence of Mr. Kushi's dynamic presence, agreed without hesitation. "We are very strong people."

The next question was directed to me. "How do you feel now?"

My answer came unhesitatingly, "Very, very happy, Mr. Kushi."

The smile on his face told me he already knew the answer before he asked the question.

"Then please tell me about your illness."

Chronologically, I related everything that happened since January 13th 1987 when I was diagnosed with Stage IV ovarian cancer. He listened quietly, not interrupting my testimony. Even Dragomir's fluent translating left that intimate moment undisturbed.

"Good," he said, after hearing my story. "Please take your coat off. And your watch, please. And your necklace. Please do not wear them."

He took my pulse, touched my palms, examined my shoulders and spine, looked into my eyes, at my tongue and checked my feet.

"Very good," he said. "It will be very difficult. But in one year you will be well."

I glanced at Bosko. Tears stained his cheeks. I felt like hugging Mr. Kushi for the kind way he told me. It sounded reasonable and simple. Truth was staring me in the face. Instead, I hugged Bosko.

"Let's design your diet and then talk about a new way of life."

His words sounded like: "Let's dance. Let's play. Let's have fun as you journey on the river of life."

Now it was our turn to listen. And listen we did, for an hour-and-a half. A new diet was prescribed. It sounded like a "No, no diet." *Avoid this, avoid that.* He recited my "black list": no meat, chicken, dairy and dairy products, eggs, sugar, tropical fruit, raw fruit, artificial sweeteners, coffee, alcohol, soft drinks, food colors, canned food, and raw vegetables. No nightshade vegetables: tomato, potato, egg plant, bell peppers and no high potassium vegetables with oxalic acid, such as spinach.

There went my delicious traditional Yugoslav cuisine.

My daily diet consisted of 50% whole grains, 5% protein; 5% seaweed, 25 – 45% vegetables, *miso* soup once a day, 2% pickles and every ten days one half cup of cooked fruit. For daily seasoning I could use 1/2 teaspoon *miso*. I also could use one teaspoon *shoyu* soy sauce in one dish per meal. A special medicinal pickled *umeboshi plum* was recommended four times per week. Four times a week in pressed salad I could have one teaspoon of vinegar obtained from processing those plums. In my case, sea salt was prohibited for four months. Grains were to be cooked with *kombu* seaweed and one-half teaspoon *gomashio* was to be sprinkled over cooked grains.

One cup of whole grains to be served with each meal. The primary grain should be 80% short grain brown rice, combined with 20% of other grains; whole wheat; rye; *hato mugi,* and whole oats. Secondary grain was whole barley; the third, millet. In summer I could eat fresh corn daily and long grain brown rice two or three times a week. Food must be whole and organic. No processed or refined foods for six months. That included sourdough bread, whole wheat pasta, and pastries. The only raw vegetables allowed were pressed, fermented salad. Fermenting preserves enzymes. Further recommendations were: no oil for four months, no fish for six months.

Protein was limited. I could have only one-half cup daily of medicinal beans: *azuki,* garbanzos (chickpeas), dark green lentils, black soybeans and once a week, *tempeh* and *tofu,* a 2" x 2" piece of each. Before each meal, I was to have 2 slices of *daikon radish* pickled in rice bran and sea salt.

He suggested certain internal and external home remedies to be incorporated into my recovery plan. (See Appendix B) These help the body eliminate excess fat, mucus and toxins without traumatic side effects. *Ume-Sho-kuzu drink* was recommended four times a week to strengthen digestion, restore energy, improve intestinal condition, and deal with stomach problems.

Carrot/daikon drink was to be taken every other day for two months. This drink helps dissolve solidified fat deposits existing deep within the body.

"We don't have daikon radish in our country. If I buy fresh daikon radish here, how long will it remain fresh?" I wondered.

"Daikon will last two weeks. If you can't find it use black radish which is common in your country. It has similar medicinal effects."

"I'll buy some seeds and grow them in my garden," I promised myself out loud.

"Very good," Mr. Kushi seemed pleased.

Another beneficial remedy is *Sweet vegetable drink.* Mr. Kushi developed this is to help overcome the effect of long term eating of chicken, eggs, and cheese leading to hypoglycemia or chronic low blood sugar. This drink softens tightness caused by heavy animal food consumption and relaxes the body. It is especially beneficial for softening the pancreas and stabilizes blood sugar levels.

Azuki bean and *black soybean tea* were recommended three times a week for proper regulation of kidney and urinary functions and for smooth bowel movement.

'Discharge' is the term used in macrobiotics to describe the process by which the body eliminates fat, mucus and toxins. Anticipating my discharge, Mr. Kushi recommended that I drink dried *shiitake mushroom tea* for two months. This tea is traditionally used to reduce fever, dissolve animal quality fat and relax a contracted or tense condition. In case of high fever, he suggested *daikon drink number. 1,* to be taken raw with hot *bancha tea.*

Then he outlined my new macrobiotic lifestyle and suggested home care. (See Appendix B for Lifestyle Suggestions and Home Care.)

Whew! That was a lot! It seemed easier to continue bad habits than start good ones. But I was ready and willing, with no negative comment. I knew something was wrong with my previous way of life and my place in nature. Day after day, I had been going without sunshine or daylight, working under fluorescent lights, feeling guilty for not having time to enjoy life. My only exercise had been washing eighteen windows in my house. That's why all those toxins, fat and mucus were trapped in my body, becoming solidified tumors.

We talked about an ill person's attitude. It's important to forgive and to be forgiven. Accept everything with unlimited joy and gratitude, expressing thankfulness for everything and to everyone. Be prepared to understand and accept whatever happens. Have faith in what you are doing. Educate yourself through macrobiotics.

We understood from Dragomir that Mr. Kushi usually didn't spend so much time talking about the philosophical aspects of macrobiotics. Did he sense our commitment and dedication? I knew then what he already knew. I would follow his instructions unerringly.

Everything fell into place as if it was meant to be. I was ready. Bosko was ready. Mr. Kushi reawakened our natural, inherent health consciousness. How had we lost our compass for natural living? How did we lose our roots? Look, we just found them again!

That's why our teacher's suggestion to sing a happy song every day didn't sound silly to us. I couldn't remember the last time I sang a happy song. What defies explanation is that for the last eleven years, the monitor control in my office at the radio station had been piping in music every day! Come to think of it, I couldn't remember words to even one song. How could that happen? It sounded like my life up until then was a tragedy interspersed with a picnic here and there. From now on, I intended to live a better quality life; to silence death which was mocking me to my face.

Does that sound like the Phoenix in Egyptian mythology? It's the story of a beautiful lone bird that lives in the Arabian desert for 600 years. It sets itself on fire, only to rise anew from the ashes to start another long life; a symbol of immortality.

As Dragomir was consulting with Mr. Kushi, I shared this thought with Bosko, "Doesn't my life sound like the story of the mythological Phoenix?" My lips tenderly touched his cheek. Wow! How wondrous! That someone so sick could feel so contented.

Drawing me close, he playfully whispered in my ear, "Don't worry. I will watch you very carefully, so you won't burn your wings."

"See you next year," we said to Mr. Kushi. I knew then that I would live to do just that!

He wished us all the best and a safe trip home. Leaving the Institute, hope and faith took charge of my healing.

Emerging from the subway I triumphantly reminded Bosko, "Today is exactly one month since my doctor's prognosis of two months to live. I feel better than ever. I feel fantastic; no pain in my body. I sleep well. My appetite is excellent. My happiness transcends all understanding. How could cancer possibly survive in my body?"

Bosko was thrilled with my new perspective. "From now on, let's not use the word 'cancer.' Let's adopt Mr. Kushi's term, 'condition.'"

Raising my arms skyward and lifting my head with an expression of thanks, I exclaimed, "I love my life! My life is like the Phoenix!"

Chapter 9

Macrobiotics in Yugoslavia

The Phoenix Rises

Next morning we arrived at Logan Airport with six suitcases full of food, hopefully enough for six months, and another two of clothes and diapers. Our luggage was stuffed with organic grains, beans, seaweed, miso paste, soy sauce, sea salt, all kinds of vinegar, kitchen utensils, lots of seeds, and surprises for our children. We were very eager to succeed.

Sinking more comfortably into my seat, I gazed out the window. Here I am entering the universe… uninvited! Am I a lawbreaker? Are we intruders? What are we doing here? How long will the universe tolerate this? Are we breaking universal laws? Fear enveloped me. Man insolently disobeys universal order, the eternal law of God. Ignoring proof to the contrary, without permission or authority he boldly takes it all for granted. Shamelessly, he's determined to go the limit, believing he will never be held accountable. I'm ready for confession!

Lightning shivers through my body, chilling me to the bone. Bosko gently covers me with a blanket as I rest my head against the seat. I'm warm and safe. I escape into meditation. Faint echoes whisper from the soft, white, cushiony clouds, *"We are one. Love is the only energy of the One. Let her bless you and heal you."* It sounds unreal, a fantasy, but I accept the logic and simplicity of that message. Birds, plants, animals and everything moving on this planet obey universal law… except man. Consuming sun, air, water, they balance themselves with nature's constant changes. My newly learned perspective on life arouses within me a reawakening and deeper respect for the powerful forces that make this happen. Everything begins to make more sense. The universal Law of Change — or yin and yang — is the basic principle of life. Every phenomena is the bringing together of these two forces; such as day and night, hot and cold, wet and dry, in varying combinations and proportions. Everything is relative, nothing is neutral in the river of life — which we call our world.

Those twenty hours passed like the blink of an eye. Deplaning in Belgrade, our loved ones greeted us with bouquets of flowers and hugs amidst tears. Srdjan and Yelena were crying for joy. At home, exactly like our farewell, our warm-hearted family, friends and neighbors welcomed us and took away our tiredness. The kids and Ratka couldn't wait for us to open the suitcases. Yelena liked macrobiotic goodies, candies, cookies and muffins. Srdjan admired his new look, posturing in front of the mirror with his new sweatshirt and Nikes. Rummaging through the suitcases, Ratka opened the ones with food first. With each one, she let out a whoop. Holding for the first time things she had previously only read about.

"Azuki beans! These cute little burgundy reds. Nigari! We can make our own tofu. Koji! Kids, we're going to make amasake, a delicious rice dessert."

The kids looked at each other, wondering curiously, "What's the big deal? What's she getting so excited about?"

Zlata, my sister-in-law, started putting food in jars and labelling them. They stayed up most of the night and decided that Ratka would stay two more weeks until I got stronger. During her last week, she would teach Zlata how to cook, assuming that was enough time for me to be taking care of myself. Next evening Ratka, Zlata and Bosko started working on a very important assignment: translating the philosophy, consultation list and recipes from *The Cancer Prevention Cookbook*. They prepared my menu for the next day. (See Appendix B for Menu)

Found among those translated pages were these forgotten truisms. Human motion is a part of the ceaseless movement of the universe. When humans are in harmony with the universe, our world is suffused with sublime beauty and supreme peace. When they are not in harmony, chaos and confusion result. Our happiness depends upon our judgment. Illness or health, intelligence or foolishness, piety or vice, depend upon our judgment. Judgment develops upward toward perfection.

Absolute and universal love embraces everything and turns every antagonism into complementarism. Judgment of thought, moral judgment. There are many ways to make a happy life. One of the most powerful is family life. The creation of a healthy family — a warm, bright family — is the resting place of the soul, the root of life and the spine of vitality. If a household is gloomy, sad and cold, life is so miserable we're bound to search elsewhere for joy, pleasure and comfort. Children are the center of our life. Life goes on from day to day. Too often we forget that our purpose as human beings is to create beautiful, healthy offspring and to secure a naturally healthy life for future generations. A happy and healthy family is the soil of culture. We come from the soil! We are part of the soil! The family has always been a primary consideration in traditional culture. Now was the time for our family to put this into practice.

My new life regimen began February 28th, 1987. Each rule written by Mr. Kushi was to be followed precisely. This was my daily schedule:

5:30 a.m.	Rise, scrub body with hot ginger towel
6:00 — 6:30 a.m.	Yoga, Do-In (self massage)
6:30 — 7 a.m.	Visualization
7:00 — 7:15 a.m.	Preparing children for school
7:15 — 8 a.m.	Preparing breakfast
8:00 — 9 a.m.	Breakfast, chewing each bite 200 times
9:00 — 9:30 a.m.	Walk — snack, medicinal drink
9:30 — Noon	Cooking lunch
Noon — 1 p.m.	Lunch, chewing each mouthful 200 times
1:00 — 1:30 p.m.	Walk, snack, medicinal drink
1:30 — 3:30 p.m.	Time for reading macrobiotic and other books Time with family
3:30 — 5:30 p.m.	Cooking dinner
5:30 — 6:30 p.m.	Dinner, chewing each mouthful 200 times
6:30 — 7 p.m.	Walk, snack, medicinal drink
6:30 — 9:30 p.m.	Time with family, education, scrubbing body with hot towel dipped in hot water, followed with 17 second shower
10:00 p.m.	Bedtime — prayers with family

After the second week, living by this regime, my body started to respond. It was difficult to walk, my legs were very heavy, but nothing stopped me from exercising faithfully. I knew the discomfort meant my body was beginning to release accumulated poisons.

My family adapted well and adjusted to our new lifestyle. Yelena was attached to my skirt; my right hand 'man', my helper, from the moment I opened my eyes until day's end. Her innocent, pure spirit infused me with energy for healing. After finishing homework, Srdjan helped with clean up and dishes. He was chef-in-charge of gomashio. Bosko's job was to wash dishes and take me for a walk. Faithfully practising this routine brought astonishing results: asthma, hernia, parasites, hemorrhoids — all these were history.

Spring is my time of the year. Its birth always makes me feel a host of conflicting emotions swelling within my chest and crucifying my soul. Waves of intense emotions give me the strength to live and choose the most exciting moments in life. In spring, I am intensely drawn toward nature. Only then, in this pure, untouched natural paradise, do I feel balanced. Now my family went to that paradise almost every weekend. That was our inseparable relationship with nature.

Our spiritual life drastically changed. We started believing in the holy power of the One. We accepted the reality that we are not only responsible for our destiny but we create it. Some power exists in the universe. We believed in that power and expressed our gratitude in our prayers. We became closer to one another, more patient with one another and believed completely in what we were doing.

I watched my loved ones becoming stronger and happier, but not me. I was going through tremendous physical and emotional cleansing. Every fifteen days, my body would quiver violently, burning with a high fever. I learned to be prepared. The first time it happened was lunch-time. I started feeling chills, my body started shaking, goose bumps appeared. Ratka was there. She prepared a drink made of grated daikon with hot bancha tea. After that, I would hasten to prepare a plaster made with tofu and green cabbage. We were supposed to use leafy greens but in March we didn't have any. Cabbage worked just as well.

By the time we had prepared everything, the fever started galloping like a stampede through my body. Before I became delirious, I took my medicinal drink and applied the plaster directly on my abdomen. The attack lasted about thirty minutes. Thereafter I'd resume my duties in the kitchen.

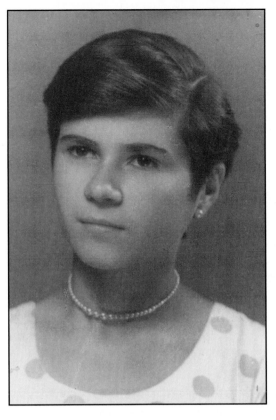

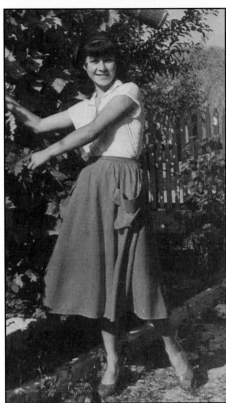

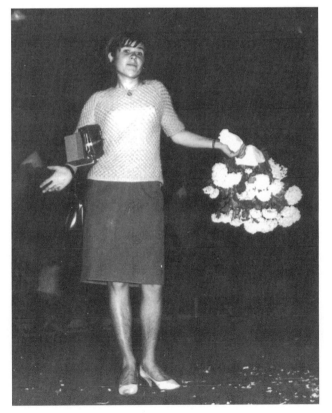

top left
Mina at age 13

top right
Mina in the village of her birth, Elemir, Yugoslavia, at age 18

bottom left
Mina receives gifts as a thank you for conducting a national ceremony to celebrate the birthday of President Tito and Yougoslavia's *Day of Youth*

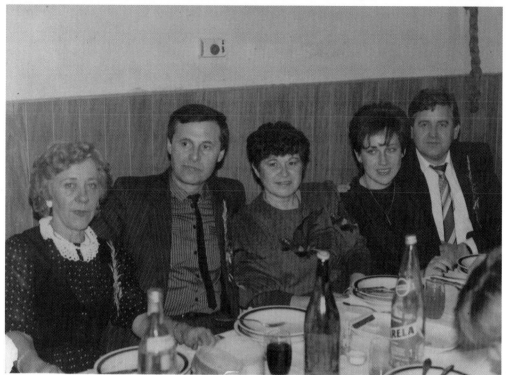

Mina, with her husband Bosko and friends, 7 months prior to her diagnosis with ovarian cancer. Notice the signs of illness in her puffy face. (1986)

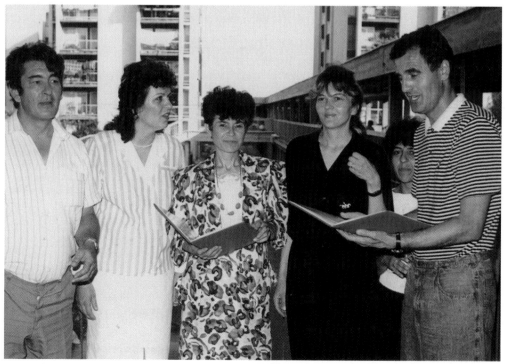

In 1987, Mina was awarded the prestigious
Truth Award for Journalism recognizing her work in the media

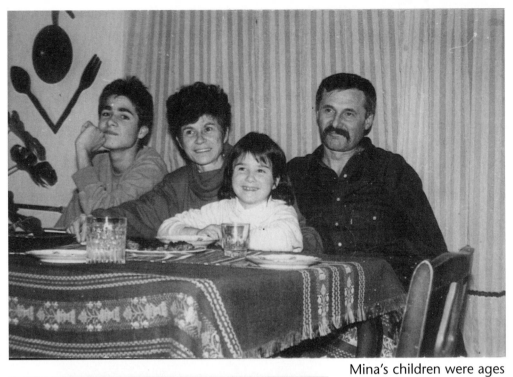

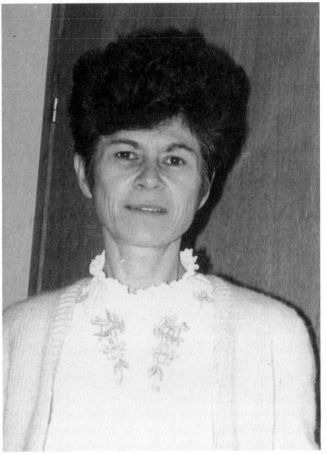

Mina's children were ages 5 and 15 when faced with the prospect of losing their mother to cancer. Pictured here in 1987, the Dobic family was packing suitcases for their journey to the United States to study for 1 year at the Kushi Institute.

After having lost 59 pounds of toxin and excess, Mina began to regain healthy pounds. (1987)

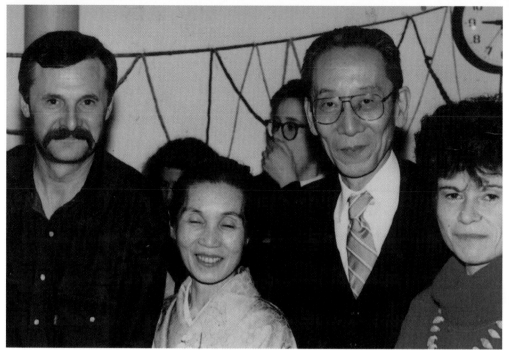

Celebrating the Chinese New year at the Kushi Institute in Boston with her teachers, Michio and Aveline Kushi, and husband Bosko (spring 1988). Mina was now cancer-free!

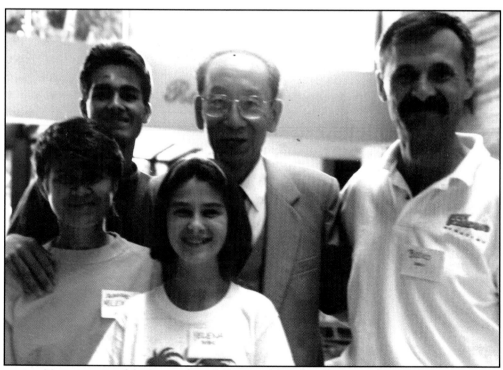

Now a macrobiotic teacher, Mina and her family attends many conferences and lectures by Michio Kushi, including this gathering in Palm Springs, Califormia, in 1991.

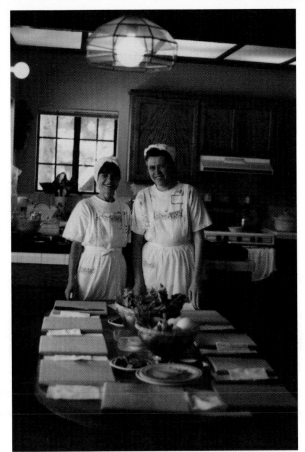

Mina and her friend Bozica Furesh from Croatia, teaching cooking classes at Mina's retreat in Big Bear, California. (1994)

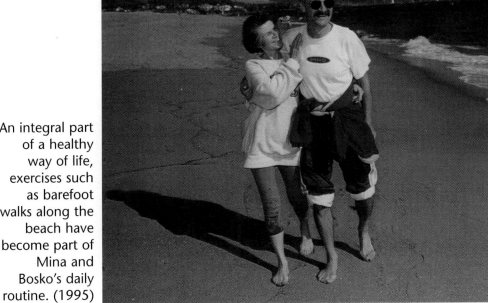

An integral part of a healthy way of life, exercises such as barefoot walks along the beach have become part of Mina and Bosko's daily routine. (1995)

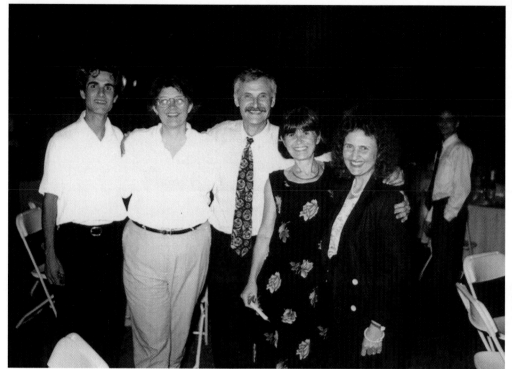

Mina has also taken an active role in fund-raising activities to support the collection on the *History of Macrobiotics* at the National Museum of American History at the Smithonian Institution. Pictured from left are Srdjan Dobic, Dr Katherine Ott, Bosko, Mina and Chris Akbar. (1997)

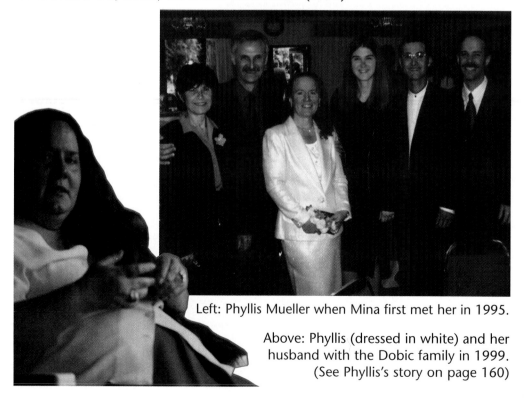

Left: Phyllis Mueller when Mina first met her in 1995.

Above: Phyllis (dressed in white) and her husband with the Dobic family in 1999.
(See Phyllis's story on page 160)

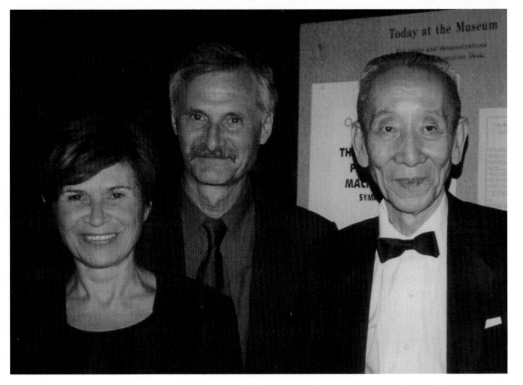

June 9, 1999: Mina, Bosko and their teacher Michio Kushi at the
National Museum of American History of the Smithonian Institution
in Washington DC, for the grand opening on the
History of Macrobiotics and Alternative and Complementary Health Practice.

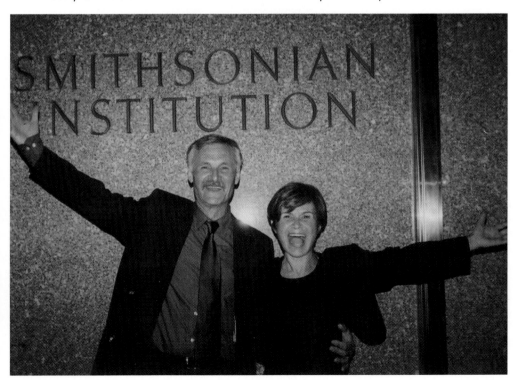

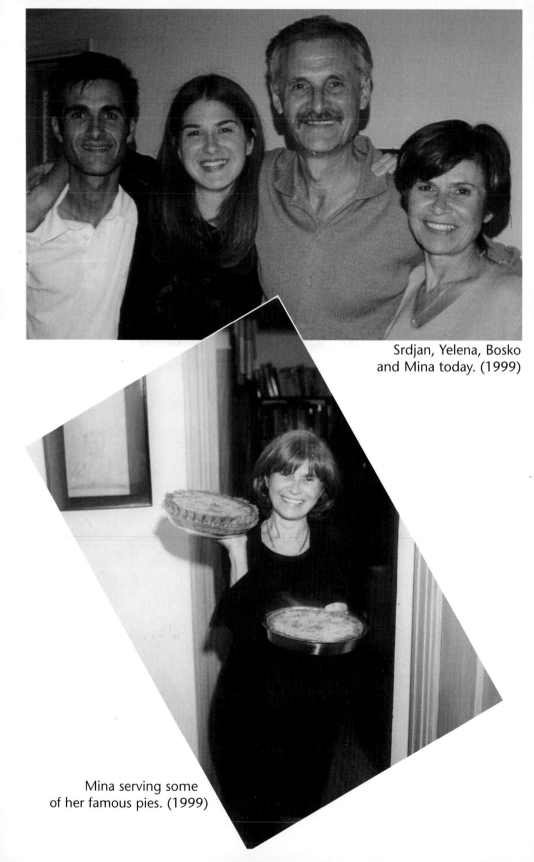

Srdjan, Yelena, Bosko
and Mina today. (1999)

Mina serving some
of her famous pies. (1999)

My 179 pound figure started melting, while my emotional and spiritual persona thrived. There were times when the food didn't taste good. We had learned at the Boston seminar that if you prepare your own food, putting your energy in it, your own energy is doubled. Now my conscience began prodding me to take over the cooking. Positive thoughts put positive energy in the food; because you're doing it for all the right reasons. Positive thoughts heal.

Besides, it was time for Ratka to leave. I was grateful for all she had done, but not overcome with sadness. I accepted the prospect ahead, understanding that it was time for me to take charge. Except that I couldn't stand on my feet. Bosko found a wheelchair and mounted my cutting board on it. All day long I traveled from refrigerator to sink, sink to stove, stove to dining table.

I had to ask Zlata to help me for one more week. After ten days, I didn't need the wheelchair anymore. Zlata was not only a great help, she was my guardian angel. She and Bosko were marvelous company. We had the best of times. They made my recovery easier. They worked very hard, cooking, cleaning, translating, and entertaining. The spirit in our home was one of joy, understanding and happiness.

Snow started melting from the rooftops and spring was knocking on the door. I stopped my sixty-day count down — the two month deadline for my demise had passed. When Zlata left I worked all day long, sometimes from 6 a.m. to 7 p.m. I never omitted one thing from my daily schedule, even though my energy was short. If I stopped moving, I'd never get rid of toxins and stagnation. I pushed myself to do all the exercises on my program. Sometimes tearfully. My body was rusty and inflexible but with each passing day I got better. In three months I lost 59 pounds. Reduced to skin and bones. My special "bagel" cushion became my constant companion. If I forgot it, my bones would cut through my skin.

One Sunday lunchtime, all chewing religiously, Yelena broke the silence. Her voice sad, in a mournful tone she blurted out, "Mommy, I'm so afraid of you. You look like a skeleton."

Bosko and Srdjan started criticizing her. I stopped them short. "Don't worry, my Sunshine, very soon I'll start gaining weight. A couple more weeks and your mommy is going to look better, more beautiful, and you're going to love me more."

"No. I'm not going to love you more, because I already love you the most!"

We all loved the food, even though I cooked the same things over and over for six months. For the first couple of months we were constantly hungry. Wherever we went, we took tons of food. Bosko worried because, despite my constant eating, I was continuing to loose weight. So he called the Kushi Institute to inquire about that. The answer was a reminder of the known rule. Chew, chew, chew!

Mr. Kushi said emphatically, "Please tell your wife she's eating too much food. She's feeding her cancer. Eat less. Chew more."

Thereafter, the amount of food on my smaller plate was reduced by half. Chewing for me became a religious experience. I wasn't hungry, my energy increased, the fever stopped. I put theory into practice!

During the first few months the elimination of accumulated excesses was very heavy. I used twice as many baby diapers as before. Four months later, oil and bread were added to my menu and I gained some healthy weight. I started riding my bike one mile to the outskirts of the city, and singing jubilantly as I walked barefoot through the cornfields. Enjoying the frisky corn leaves that gently touched my face, arms and legs, I felt more closely connected with the universe. Words alone cannot describe my inner gladness.

Oftentimes on my way home, I'd pick some wild flowers to place as offerings on friends' graves. I dropped by the cemetery to challenge death and weld my fate to macrobiotics, trying to relieve an inner conflict. Offering apologies that no requiem would be said for me. Saddened by the realization they had not discovered the secret for long life. "Life is play. The better you play, the longer you live." I was... I am a talented player!

Three months had passed since this healing journey began. In my kitchen, I was my own doctor. Family and friends saw a transformation happen before their eyes. They didn't understand how, so all they could do was worry. I'd been telling them about my symptoms, my good and bad discharges — pain, fever, sore throat, runny nose. I welcomed them as a sign of healing. They listened but couldn't figure out why the healing. They were confused. They wondered why a person having all those symptoms wouldn't go to a doctor for antibiotics, injections or medication? Yet I'd already tried that route.

Doctors crossed me off long ago. What could they possibly say except, "That's cancer; it's spreading. You're getting worse." I had these conditions for the first four months because the natural cycle for the exchange of new blood is 120 days.

The first week of spring, when the steam rises from mother earth, we started gardening. It was a magnificent day. Again family, friends, neighbors came to help. The hardest work was transplanting the rose bushes from the back to the front yard so we'd have a place to grow our own vegetables. We prepared the soil with organic compost and planted organic seeds to ensure the best health. Soon we would grow vegetables in the ground rather than in pots on the sunny side inside the house. We celebrated with the spirit inherent in the maxim, "From one grain, ten thousand grains."

Something interesting happened. After working only an hour-and-a-half, perspiration started dripping from our friends' foreheads and they became short of breath. They needed to take a break and asked for water. Some wondered out loud, "Mina, how come you and Bosko aren't perspiring? You don't even look tired."

Taking my professional teaching pose: "This food has more energy than toxins and it's very easy to digest. We don't have a problem with body odor any more because we don't eat meat or sugar. Our back yard is going to produce the energy necessary for our good health. Thank you all for helping prepare our soil. From that soil and these seeds we'll get our vitamins, minerals, calcium and everything else necessary for optimal health."

Less than four weeks later, we were able to make our first miso soup with fresh vegetables from our garden — red radishes with tops, scallions and parsley. That was the most delicious soup we ever ate.

Our garden was magical, a spiritual place. Working in the garden is one of the best forms of exercise and healing. That little energized spot in our backyard became a wonderland for Yelena and her friends. They quietly tiptoed into the garden, plucked baby carrots or tiny red radishes, dusted them off on their skirts and gingerly gobbled them up as they ran out giggling. Those munchkins gave me so many pleasurable moments, yet they never knew I was watching. When my kitchen window was open and one of her friends started to complain about radishes being too hot, I overheard Yelena whispering with her mouth full, "Just chew. This is very good to clean the fat from your body." Here we go. Another macrobiotic teacher. Like mother, like daughter.

Fifty percent of our diet consisted of vegetables which we grew in our garden. Some of the food we imported from "Yin and Yang — Natur — Kost" health food in Graz, Austria. Father supplied legumes from his garden. Grains we got in packages from all over the country. During a TV interview, I discussed the difficulty of obtaining organic grains. Shortly thereafter, farmers started shipping us organic grains. We got enough for the next six months. From Bosnia, we received rye; from Croatia, barley; from Macedonia, 100 pounds of short grain brown rice, 50 pounds of chickpeas.

Excitedly, I mentioned that in just two more months, I could eat my first fish in six months! Someone surprised us with a fresh caught halibut which arrived exactly on time, the last week of the sixth month. That was a long trip for the fish, it traveled over 600 miles from the Croatian part of the Adriatic Coast. That was a very valuable gift. The only fish we could get in our part of the country was fresh water fish. We had a fish feast which we shared with our neighbors. Some people might not understand how we could make such a celebration over a fish but this event gave meaning to our goal. We had more fun than gypsies. Bosko played the accordion all night long. We sang longer and louder than usual. Nobody cared, they were having too much fun.

These charitable gifts represented tremendous savings. It enabled us to stretch our financial resources. Whatever happened in those last six months we accepted as positive. Anything negative we accepted as part of the transition. People in my country were very caring, supportive and human. That gave me reason to rejoice all the more. I was a different person with a new perspective which enabled me to take the next step: choosing to teach macrobiotics.

Practising macrobiotics doesn't deprive us of anything others enjoy. On the contrary, we simply exchange one lifestyle for a better one. Month by month, this lifestyle gradually became a pleasant habit.

Having experienced the elan of macrobiotic living, we were overflowing with a desire to share it with others. We warned everybody in sight that the food they were eating was harmful. (The same food we'd been eating a short while before.) We warned them of dire consequences if they didn't immediately change.

I recalled the summer of 1986 — a year prior to my being diagnosed with cancer. We were spending a holiday with Ratka, Andrija and their children on the Mediterranean coast. Ratka had suggested preparing macrobiotic food for the entire ten days of our holiday. I agreed. Bosko and Andrija took ham, cheese and bacon "just in case." The entire ten days Ratka and I ate macrobiotic food. Our carnivorous husbands called it "canary food." It couldn't, they said, provide them with enough energy to swim. They ate meat for breakfast, lunch and dinner. It frequently caused headaches. They popped pills endlessly. The negative energy generated led to internecine conflict. We ladies expected their livers to explode any minute.

After the vacation, I decided to join Ratka and continue eating macrobiotic food. Notwithstanding her training as an allopathic pediatrician which had given her a different view of degenerative disease, she recognized that food can both cause and heal dis-ease. Unbeknownst to me, she recognized the early symptoms of cancer and urged me to adopt macrobiotics. I was too dedicated to my career to make the necessary changes in my way of life. Out of ignorance, I did it for two weeks and quit. Looking back with 20-20 hindsight, I realize the cancer might never have developed if I'd listened to my friend. It took a cosmic kick in the "bottom" to awaken me. Cancer was my teacher and my savior.

From day one, I excitedly shared my discovery with others. As the old saying goes, I was "talking against the wind." People are in a hypnotic state of somnolence, unable to accept the simplicity of natural healing.

Today, eleven years later, I am glad I shared my discovery with others. "Macrobiotics" means long life. Perhaps time and patience will help people realize what I'd experienced.

With the change of seasons, methods of cooking changed. In summer, we ate less, cooking took less time. Our metabolism changed and our body chemistry balanced. I gained 25 pounds over the next six months. My energy doubled. I remained calm and relaxed. The only discharge I still had was vaginal and my use of diapers was down to 3 or 4 a day.

In early summer we heard Michio Kushi would conduct a Macrobiotic Summer Camp in Switzerland. We scheduled an appointment. Carrying our small mobile kitchen and groceries, we arrived after traveling two days. Another red letter day.

At midnight we met with Mr. Kushi for my first follow up consultation. After a brief examination he said, "Good. Very good job. Your recovery will take only two more months."

Actually I had anticipated such a diagnosis. During the previous two months, for the first time in my life, I had felt completely whole. I was eating to live, not living to eat.

Mr. Kushi now changed my diet. I was to cook with a higher flame for less time. Grains, beans and sea vegetables would be cooked separately; then mixed with blanched, quick steamed or boiled vegetables to create delicious summer salads. The kids were thrilled. Srdjan's favorite salad was marinated tempeh with sea vegetables and spring greens.

Bosko loved fish with vegetables and red sauce (similar to marinara sauce), but made with carrots, onion, celery and *umeboshi* plum. Yelena's favorite meal was *seitan gravy* and *millet mashed potatoes*. According to the new menu, I could have melon, watermelon and fruit *kanten* twice a week. Boiled corn on the cob with umeboshi paste was our favorite snack. What was happening now was somehow easier and more spontaneous.

Questions I asked myself while praying were: Am I,

- eating today in harmony with my environment?

- thinking of my parents, relatives, teachers, and elders with love and respect?

- happily greeting everyone today and expressing an interest in their life?

- contemplating the sky, the trees, and the flowers and marveling at the wonders of nature?

- thanking everyone and appreciating everything I experience today?

- performing my tasks faithfully and thereby contributing to a more peaceful world?

This spiritual frame of mind surrounded me with peace.

January 13th 1988 marked one year since my diagnosis. I wanted another follow up consultation with Mr. Kushi. Once again, friends and relatives came to our aid. Within a week they had raised the necessary finances.

This trip to Boston was more like a vacation. We were eager to get there. The city was hidden beneath a satiny white blanket of snow. We revisited Barbara's home. She greeted us warmly. Everything went smoothly. Familiar paths took us back to Open Sesame restaurant. Miso soup warmed our hearts. Dragomir and Seka were as delighted to see us as we to see them.

We had plenty of time to see Boston, a city possessed of a European look and spirit. We bubbled with enthusiasm upon visiting Cambridge. Youth swarmed through Cambridge Square in front of Harvard University. We were bathed and penetrated by powerful vibrations — literally!

I recalled the description of Harvard as the "home bastion of science, world-renowned and highly esteemed intelligence." How profoundly would this world be changed if this army of youth were to become health conscious? Is that possible? I recalled the old tag, times are changed and we are changing in them. Wouldn't a good macrobiotic restaurant in Cambridge Square be a start? (Ten years later a part of that dream became reality. Masao's Kitchen, a small macrobiotic restaurant, is now an oasis of healthy food for many university students.)

My consultation was scheduled for January 27th. It was so cold, our hands stuck to icy doorknobs. This time Mr. Kushi welcomed us as old friends. We were flattered. My examination lasted fifteen minutes. He asked me to take off my jacket, shoes and socks. I was embarrassed taking off five layers of clothing. Three slips, two skirts, two pairs of slacks. There I was standing in my one piece, ankle length jumpsuit. A mountain of clothes beside me. Boy, was I skinny! During the examination I anticipated the results, "Very good, very good, excellent, good job."

Mr. Kushi was bending down, checking my feet. Then he stood up extended his hand toward me and said simply without pomp, "Congratulations. You are cancer free."

Yes! The Phoenix Rises!

It was as if he had given me a "green card". Easter bells rang in my soul. I heard a message coined in Roman times: the most wonderful thing is when a man overcomes himself.

Bosko couldn't believe his ears. We struggled to remain calm. I relished my dietary changes: bread three times a week, pasta three or four times a week, rice with vegetables and oil, sesame seed butter, carrot and apple juice.

Sadness washed over me as I left the Kushi Institute. I wanted to stay forever. I promised myself out loud: "I'll be back here to study."

Bosko concurred, "That could be possible."

Back at our hotel we couldn't contain our joy. We had to share it with our friends. We phoned Radio Station Indjija. My recovery was broadcast by the Yugoslav national media. They carried my voice live: "Nature has healed my cancer." A few minutes later they called me back. My colleagues were holding a party to celebrate my recovery. From all over Yugoslavia relatives and friends were celebrating, "Mina is alive."

Four days later, March 17th, we flew home.

In April 1988 I returned to public life. But with a more worthwhile and common goal — helping people and the planet to recover. A radio program was the most effective way to awaken mass health consciousness. I asked for and received a four hour daily program: "Healthy Human Environment Prevents Illness." It met with overwhelming interest. Live interviews were conducted with health conscious citizens: farmers, artists, actors, teachers, workers, professors, athletes, scientists, government officials.

Television again got interested in the subject. Newspaper articles appeared: "Yugoslav female journalist wins fight against cancer with macrobiotics." The media again invaded our home for interviews. Very often programs were broadcast from there, due to my busy schedule. Public interest mounted. Our telephone rang constantly. Our home became the Balkan macrobiotic institute.

On their way to European countries, people came to me first for advice on what foods to buy and where to get them. On their way back, they came for further assistance in translating labels. At times, I even did the labelling for them.

In early 1988, interest in macrobiotics had increased in Belgrade, Zagreb, capital of Croatia, and Novi Sad, Vojvodina province. I received invitations for seminars, lectures, and sessions. Doctor Karmensita Maskarel Berich, an esteemed pathophysiologist, organized a lecture for her medical colleagues on macrobiotics. I was invited as guest lecturer to explain how food acted as medicine in my case. It was a very successful seminar. Next day the most widely read national newspaper printed a front page article entitled, "Doctor, is my illness caused by the food I eat?"

By then macrobiotic seminars had started in Belgrade and the interest was overwhelming. Zlatko Pejic, a Croatian macrobiotic leader, held seminars throughout the country. That marked the beginning of a movement to return to traditional, natural food. On many occasions I was invited as a guest or lecturer.

We were deluged by a steady flow of the sick. Our home became a mecca for the hopelessly ill. We were being invaded by the helpless and needy, powerless to satisfy their requirements. We couldn't help them because our knowledge wasn't enough. Those events greatly influenced our later decision to return to Boston and continue our studies at the Kushi Institute.

In 1988 my family and friends decided to arrange a macrobiotic seminar and invite Mr. Kushi to come to Yugoslavia. His lectures were advertised extensively on radio and TV. A series of three lectures were scheduled, two in Belgrade and one in Zagreb, capital of Croatia. Michio and his wife, Aveline Kushi came, accompanied by a few medical doctors from Europe and the U.S. who successfully incorporated macrobiotics into their practice. The first lecture was targeted toward the medical community. No one could have ever anticipated such an overwhelming response. To our amazement, over 700 medical doctors attended that lecture! I must say, Mr. Kushi was brilliant. His presentation was eagerly received and the response was positive. The second lecture, open to the general public, was attended by 2,000. The climax of his visit and his final lecture was before a packed-out audience in the huge music hall in Zagreb. Enthusiastically he stated that Yugoslavia had immense possibilities for improving its national health:

"Despite its geographical position, Yugoslavia did not keep pace with world technology movements as did the neighboring parts of the Western world. This third world eastern country didn't accept everything as fast as the rest of modern civilization did by submitting [its] lifestyle to consumer fever which resulted in pollution of [the] human environment. Possibilities for expanding macrobiotics are great. You are not even aware of what can be achieved. You have a lot of cultivated and clean land which you can use for growing biologically healthy foods. All you would have to do is pull out pages from old cook books, refresh those recipes and that would be all you need to get started."

He was talking about food quality, energy, causes and effects of unhealthy foods.

"Think about people who are ill. By spending money on unhealthy foods, in essence, they are inflicting further harm upon themselves. All those expensive products of our modern age such as chocolate, candies, biscuits, cakes, mayonnaise, creams, meat and eggs, are human killers. People become addicted to those foods which make them depressed and sick. In turn, they try to compensate for this by eating more of the same foods. People were healthier when they consumed less sugar, white flour and meat, which are in fact the biggest enemies to humans nowadays. Money created more harm than benefit to the wealthy ones, whereas the poor and modest sustained a healthier lifestyle. This is especially true if they have not used a microwave oven, which by the way, I recommend you give as a gift to your enemy."

It was obvious that people in the auditorium were taken by his speech, as they listened carefully to the true facts about human health and admired Michio Kushi's promotion of healthy life. His slogan was "to sing while you make food and at any other time, which will eventually make you happier and healthier." That was the front page title next day in newspapers and magazines. Macrobiotics made a grand entrance through a wide open door in Yugoslavia, and took a prominent position in the everyday life of many health conscious people.

At about the same time Zlatko Pejic organized a week long seminar in Croatia, with medical personnel from throughout the country. Michio Kushi lectured and Aveline Kushi conducted cooking lessons. I was fascinated by that quiet little Japanese woman in her sixties. Her fingers magically touched and shaped vegetables. Everything she did had inconceivable serenity and artful rhythm. Her cooking was art, a feast for eyes and soul.

I shall always marvel at how she could be at the same time a great mother to her children, excellent wife to an eminent philosopher, compatriot, partner and fighter for peace and human happiness, and teacher of cookery art. She is a woman of extraordinary personal qualities, a mother to a thousand other young people who came from all over the world to visit, study and live at her home.

Their visit generated an awakening… a reawakening, a kind of renaissance that rocked the entire country. Television Novi Sad conducted an interview with me which had a great influence on macrobiotic development. It was an avalanche of change. The government took the lead. Programs were initiated to start growing produce without the use of dangerous pesticides and chemicals. The Chief of Staff at the Children's Hospital eliminated dairy and chicken from the menu and substituted rice, soy products and fish. That same doctor cured himself of lung cancer with macrobiotics. In only one month in Belgrade, the macrobiotic community grew to a staggering 2,000 people! Lectures, seminars, support groups, began to spring up everywhere. Local farmers wanted to grow organic vegetables and fruit. It was altogether incredible! It was my happy privilege to be there, microphone in hand, reporting all of it — live!

At the end of his first visit, Mr. Kushi invited me and my family to come to Boston to study. We had enormous financial and moral support from our dearest friends. In four months time, we managed to collect enough money for a decent existence. We control our destiny and in the process elevate our consciousness to promote us into heroes. Such moments are usually turning points in life, transforming us into new personalities.

The die was cast! We planned to go within a year and take the children with us.

Much had to be sorted out before we left. We had to make sure that Bosko's mother was financially secure. Arrangements were made to have our dear neighbors take care of her and live in our home rent-free. Airline tickets were booked for a September 4th flight to Boston.

Chapter 10

Becket:

Training for Future Career

Finally my dream had come true. I would be studying macrobiotics with Michio and Aveline Kushi and my family was going with me. The macrobiotic leaders who came to my country made it all possible.

Another tearful but joyous sendoff by our loved ones. This time we were better prepared, having no fear or uncertainty.

Our kids were beside themselves with glee. Srdjan couldn't wait to get aboard. Aeroplanes were his fascination. Yelena was afraid of flying but once we took off she relaxed and settled in. Of course, we brought plenty of food and it was a smooth flight.

Upon arriving, we headed straight to "Anthony Town House." Barbara was very pleased to see us again. She was favorably impressed with the kids' good behavior and offered free accommodation for them. She spared no effort to make her "small pleasant European family" comfortable. We spent hours bringing her up to date with all the good things that had transpired since last we saw her.

The following afternoon we got in touch with Mr. Kushi and were dismayed to learn he wouldn't be available for five more days. We were very concerned. Why the delay? Our daily costs were: apartment: $50, food: $30. By Yugoslav standards, that was a lot of money. Concerned that the delay would cost us almost $400, I insisted Bosko explain the situation to Mr. Kushi.

Moved with compassion, Mr. Kushi arranged an earlier appointment. At first sight Kushi House in Brookline gives an impression of opulence but it is not so. Its interior furnishings are spotlessly clean, orderly, modest and cozy. The atmosphere harmonic, serene and peaceful.

Mr. Kushi greeted us warmly. We sank down comfortably into our chairs, feeling welcome and relaxed.

"What is your purpose for coming to America?" he wanted to know.

"I am here to give support to my wife in every respect and to learn about macrobiotics," Bosko replied quickly and without hesitation.

"My dream is to study macrobiotics, help those in need, and teach healthy people how to prevent illness," Bosko easily translated for me.

"And what would you like to do here," Mr. Kushi asked Srdjan, meeting eye to eye.

Coming from a conservative society, we're not accustomed to giving decision-making freedom to children. Therefore, to ask a child such a question seemed inappropriate. How could a 16-year-old possibly be expected to know what decision to make for his destiny? Especially having just arrived in a foreign country?

Bosko quickly replied, "We want Srdjan to continue high school but we don't know how or where."

Mr. Kushi turned to Srdjan again. "But what would you like to do young man?"

"I would like to learn macrobiotics here in Boston," was Srdjan's confident reply, as if feeling Mr. Kushi's support.

"Now we know," concluded Mr. Kushi. "Mr. Dobic, you, your wife and daughter can study at the Macrobiotic Institute in Becket which is in the Berkshire Mountains about 230 miles away."

"You, Srdjan," pronouncing his name easily, "will be able to study macrobiotics here in Boston at the Kushi Institute and live with us in our home. Costs of living and education will be arranged as a work exchange."

"Tonight you can all sleep here so you don't have to pay for hotel accommodations but tomorrow our agreement will go into effect. Welcome."

Mr. Kushi had turned another page in our lives. Another new beginning! One of the students took us to our room. There we spent what was to be our last night together for a long time. It was a small studio apartment with kitchenette overlooking a nearby park. An enchanting view like a healing balm that soothes the eye. My dream fulfilled as if by magical power now manifested itself. A light lost then found, essential to achieving a meaningful life.

We were exhausted. Empowered by inner joy, we offered a prayer of thankfulness for our hosts' loving acceptance. Sinking into the comfortable futon, we fell asleep cuddling and embracing one another.

Next morning, seated on floor cushions at a long, low table, we were served breakfast. The modest dining room was nearly empty. Warm greetings instantly made us feel like part of the family. Mr. and Mrs. Kushi and their young son were sitting opposite us. On either side sat two young male students, one from England, one from Israel. The room gave off a feeling of spiritual warmth.

We watched closely, careful to copy what the others were doing. We ate slowly, chewing in silence. After breakfast we were taken to the bus station for a three-hour trip to Lee, a small town twenty miles from Becket. Upon our arrival a driver would take us the rest of the way to the Kushi Institute.

Mr. Kushi turned to Srdjan and asked him if he was ready to start learning.

In his eyes there was a gleam of curiosity and without hesitation, he shot back, "I am ready right now. I can't wait."

Embracing Srdjan, we said our good-byes. Bosko and I swallowed our tears but Yelena couldn't hide hers. We didn't know how long we would be apart. We would be different people when we met again. Our close bonding love would never fade. By universal law, that same love governs us all.

Srdjan stayed in Boston while attending the Kushi Institute. For him that was a challenging adventure. Only guessing what might be ahead of us, we continued our adventure by bus. We were headed toward the Berkshire Mountains. At the bus station in Lee, a young man and woman greeted us cordially. They were modestly dressed. We noticed their surprise at seeing a whole family arriving. They would have been even more surprised had Srdjan been with us.

Our drive took us through a particularly beauteous region. Nature was busily engaged in crocheting a rich tapestry of colors for the onset of fall.

Nature was magically dominating — far, far from urban elegance subdued by the artificial inertia of growth. The day was gorgeous. The dirt road was replete with potholes. The sun pierced through tree branches, delivering a spectrum of vibrant colors. The beauty and quiet calm of the forest filled us with sublime tranquillity. Suddenly the sun set. Trees became darkened, the road long and winding. Once so self assured, suddenly self doubt grips me. Had I made the best possible choice for my family? Or had I taken advantage of their unconditional love and innocence? Will they blame me later for robbing them of their true identity? Will they accuse me of depriving them of a comfortable, easy and secure life? By one act of arrogance I have ripped our children away from all that was familiar and meaningful and dropped them into the "land of the unknown." We brought them with us because we didn't want our family separated. Now look what I have done. I have just left Srdjan with perfect strangers in a big city in a strange country.

The strength of the mountains conjured this dark vision in my soul, raising self-doubts and echoing the very thoughts conveyed by the famous Yugoslav Nobel prize winner, Ivo Andric. *It's deja vu!* I cannot push these thoughts from my memory, I find myself paraphrasing….

> *"Inexorable stern, motionless mountains looking down from cloudy heights. High and stiff sky, hard and merciless earth. No, nothing will happen. No, the mountains will not collapse. The sky will remain magnificent and cold at its altitude. A distance was slipping by, sound disappearing, colors fading away, in order to see and hear how an oppressed bloodstained heart beats.*
>
> *Where was I wandering? Where were my aspirations falling? How many times did I stumble, wandering in my mind and was wrong in life? The flame that burnt my soul down did not swallow me, but gave me strength and inspiration. The world's unrest, I did not care much about. I looked upon [it] as if I were on top of a clear height, although I was in a foggy valley. I was a silent and arrogant visitor in life."*

Yelena, asleep on my lap, changed position. Where is Srdjan sleeping now? I lovingly whispered, "Good night, sleep well." I was startled from my deep reverie. High up on the hill, houses turned white.

Maria, our new friend and driver, interrupted the silence. "Becket is down there. We will be arriving shortly."

A miniature mountain village was saying "hello" to us amidst its pleasant surroundings. Magnificent small farms, splashed everywhere, as in a fairy tale. The only significant structure in the center of the village was a general store which had everything a little village like this might need.

As the truck passed over an iron bridge, a long, roaring train passed under it. We looked down and heard the mountain river rushing underneath. Too much noise for this quiet place. Night was falling on the roof tops. As we drove down the narrow dirt road, Maria briefly described the place where we were headed. At that time it was quiet at the Kushi Institute. Only staff and a few guests were there. We stopped right in front of the main building. Here visitors stayed. It resembled an old hunting lodge with a slight edge reminiscent of oriental architecture. Here in the heart of the Berkshire Mountains, we were standing in front of a leading world macrobiotic educational center. There we were, at the center of my new universe. I thanked God for this gift and blessing!

The Kushi Institute manager Alex Jack and his wife Gale welcomed us. They seemed surprised. They showed us to our room in another building. It was in the dormitory reserved for staff and students.

A tiny room with three small futon mattresses and one closet. Walls were wood covered. The building was clean and warm inside. A tantalizing fragrance drifted from the kitchen at the end of the corridor. Our room was the second one on the way to the dining room.

We arrived at dinner time. It was like a dream. People acted as if they had known us all their lives. The meal was flavorful, prepared with fresh vegetables from their own garden. It reminded me of Thomas Mann's description in *The Magic Mountain*, but more picturesque. He wrote:

> *The mornings were very dark. They ate breakfast by the light of the artificial moons in the dining hall with its cheerfully stenciled arches. Outside was gloomy nothing, a world packed in grayish-white cotton, in foggy vapors and whirling snow that pushed up against the windowpanes. The mountains were invisible, although over time something of the nearest evergreen forest*

might come into view, heavily laden with snow, only to be quick-
ly lost in the next flurry; now and then a fir would shake off its
burden, dumping dusty white into gray. Around ten o'clock the
sun would appear like a wisp of softly illumined vapor above its
mountain, a pale spook spreading a faint shimmer of reality over
the vague, indiscernible landscape. But it all melted into a ghost-
ly delicate pallor, with no definite lines, nothing the eye could fol-
low with certainty. The contours of the peaks merged, lost in fog
and mist. Expanses of snow suffused with soft light rose in layers,
one behind another, leading your gaze into insubstantiality. And
what was probably a weakly illumined cloud clung to a cliff,
motionless, like an elongated tatter of smoke.

Around noon the sun broke halfway through, struggling to
melt the fog into blue, an attempt that fell far short of success. Yet
there was a momentary hint of blue sky and even this bit of light
was enough to release a flash of diamonds across the wide land-
scape, so oddly disfigured by its snowy adventure. Usually the
snow stopped at that hour of the day, as if for a quick survey of
what had been achieved thus far. The rare days of sunshine
seemed to serve much the same purpose — snow flurries died
down and the sun's direct glare attempted to melt the luscious,
pure surface of drifted new snow. It was a fairy tale world, child-
like and funny. Boughs of trees adorned with thick pillows, so
fluffy someone must have plumped them up; the ground a series
of humps and mounds, beneath which slinking underbrush or
outcrops of rock lay hidden; a landscape of crouching, cowering
gnomes in droll disguises — it was comic to behold, straight out of
a book of fairy tales. But if there was something roguish and fan-
tastic about the immediate vicinity through which you laborious-
ly made your way, the towering statues of snow clad Alps, gazing
down from the distance, awakened in you feelings of the sublime
and holy.

Three weeks after we arrived I included this excerpt in a letter I wrote to
my friends back home when I was trying to describe this charming place.

"Dear Compatriots,

In this intact Eden, original Nature, a human is the most sacred being on earth. A human being and Nature complement each other physically and spiritually. Humans appreciate everything they receive from Nature, rationalizing all of it materialistically. That which is received from Nature is returned with appreciation. If only you could see the plant and herb farms here at the Kushi Institute in the heart of the Berkshire Mountains in Massachusetts, where everything grows with no chemical additives, naturally and organically. How fruitful are the millet knobs and buckwheat. For the first time, I see cooperation between man and wild animals; a few chipmunks help in making natural compost for land fertilization.

This natural balance is about 150 miles away from asphalt jungles of New York. My two family members, Bosko and Yelena, found a world that lives in unity for the sake of friendship. Their hearts are filled with love and pleasure. We forget about TV, newspapers, radios, cars and busy town existence. We work in the garden, clean, sing in and around the house and cook. Everybody is happy — there are about forty of us here. We all sit at the table and enjoy all sorts of organic meals. All the vegetables picked from the garden and fields are cultivated by those who live here and all with love. I am writing this letter to you after dinner. In a while, we are going for a walk and it is still daylight at 6:30 p.m. Outside, Nature paints all possible colors under the blue sky and the sunlight.

The Berkshire heights are like a needlepoint and, at the foot of the hills, a brook serves as our water supply for the Dormitory and Main House. We all agreed to party tonight in honor of the departure of Sherman, an American writer from Israel, who came here to write a book about one peaceful world of coexistence, with no bars on it or hatred.

Only the food can make such a miracle in this crazy world. Sherman is 61-years old and already practising the macrobiotic lifestyle. He said that he had two personalities in his body: the negative ex-one and the positive present one, totally opposite. The agreement, as I said, is to have a party with macrobiotic cake and warm apple juice. We are already divided into teams. On our Slavic team, among others, are Tanjug, a journalist (telegraphic agency of Yugoslavia), Mirjana Vuckovic and a Russian woman, Zoja, an opera singer. On the International team, are Jackie from Bolivia, Monita from

Peru, Mary from Canada and Paul from Holland. The Japanese team has a head chef, Masao and Mariko Son from Hiroshima.

What a wonderful, peace-loving, brotherly world. Michio and Aveline Kushi have united people with no material interest, without the desire for prestige, right here under the roof of the International Macrobiotic Institute in the heart of the Berkshire mountains.

Could you imagine such a thing existing here in America? We feel reborn here. They are now our closest relatives, friends and colleagues. It's as if we had known each other all our lives. It seems to me that I spent 46 years looking for this kind of life. Here I am — my misfortune was a blessing in disguise.

I was extremely delighted when Mrs. Kushi called me to assist her in cooking classes during two seminars here. I was even happier when Mr. Kushi told me that I am fine healthwise and that we have a son who is going to be a good macrobiotic teacher. Srdjan will come in two weeks to visit us for four days. How long we are going to stay here, we do not know. We'll keep in touch.

Love from Mina, Bosko and kids."

Our life here at Becket started by enrolling Yelena in the second year of elementary school, which included a very intensive course in the English language. I could have used that myself. All I could say was, "Hi, how are you? I am good, thank you." Considering that my profession was linked with language, learning English was not difficult, however. I stopped calling a fork, "frog" and soon I was speaking more confidently and doing less drawing as a way of communication. Americans have a nice parlor game called "Pictionary" which I literally adored playing. This, too, helped me learn the language faster.

After only three weeks working in the kitchen as assistants to Masao the main chef, they appointed Bosko and me Head Cooks. We were given responsibility for preparing breakfast. At that time students attending the Level One Course came in from Boston. Starting at 4:30 a.m., we cooked for up to 60 people. The first morning an assistant had to help us. Everything was ready on time and served on the large dining room table.

The mornings we didn't cook, we did exercises for an hour. DO-IN, meaning self-massage, awakens vitality and promotes good blood circulation in the body. With each class, I felt my energy increasing. In my spare time I took walks. One of my favorite places was the river. As I listened to its quiet murmurings, I invited its refreshing waters to run through my veins. I wept with joy listening to low sounds of the wilderness. I regretted that so many of my mature years had been deprived of these moments. For not being spiritual enough and in tune with nature, I felt sorry for myself.

Evenings were spent in the dining room playing "Pictionary" for hours. Days and evenings were fun packed. We had gathered together from every corner of the earth with the same aim — to study the natural way of living, its philosophy on life, nourishment, cooking and to acquire tools for harmonious living.

We found many nice friends. Yelena played with kids of her age. My dearest friend was a Japanese girl, Mariko Son, a modest, good-natured, artistic soul. She was my teacher, too. I am grateful to her for my culinary art and other skills acquired for special occasions. Our life at Becket ran smoothly and joyously. We were learning every day. In one month, I acquired a knowledge of medicinal cooking and understood appropriate food balancing for specific health conditions. I knew how to balance food for a particular cancer type or other disease. I was not particularly interested in gourmet cooking. But I did learn it because I had to cook lunch and dinner. Food is served at a buffet in the dining room. One side of the table is arranged with medicinal dishes, the other side with gourmet selections. I decided to eat medicinal food for another year.

We felt constantly nurtured with wisdom, nourished with energy and transformed physically, emotionally and spiritually. We became more calm, younger looking, stronger and more healthy. Breathing in this philosophy of life meant understanding that nothing is accidental. Our world is in constant change, every second. We alone are the ultimate masters of our own reality. We have the power to choose it. We create it. We are responsible for each step on that path. The simplicity of this truth purged us from arrogance and the slightest feeling of hatred — leaving a wonderful feeling of lightness at having revisited the human soul and mind, lifting us up to a height reserved only for humans.

There were so many positive changes in our lives that I couldn't remember them all. I decided to note them down. Some of the most precious I recorded in my diary which I called simply, Becket.

September 28, 29, 30, 1988

These are the happiest days of my stay here in Becket. We are all together again. Srdjan came along with a friend for four days, to attend a special workshop at Level I and II. There were about 40 students registered. I cooked. I was beside myself with excitement. At last, I had the opportunity to cook for my son and his friends, putting all my love and good energy into their food.

I wished we could have spent more time together. Workshop classes were long and intensive. We didn't see him until after midnight. Nevertheless, I had an inner peace that brought me restful nights, fresh and happy mornings. I didn't feel at all like a person who had worked ten hours a day.

Becket, September 30, 1988

Srdjan practised yoga with his friends this morning. After an hour of practice, they went to the nearby river and swam in its icy water. Srdjan felt great. If he had done that before he became macrobiotic, he would surely have contracted a severe cold and asthma attack. Miraculously, after this adventure his lifetime of sneezing stopped completely.

In Srdjan's own words: "This day will be marked in bold letters in my life's calendar. I can clearly see how my physical condition has affected my emotional life! This medicine should be prescribed in all world cuisines, especially schools, hospitals and nursing homes. But that would be possible only if all supermarkets would start selling organic produce and other macrobiotic foods and if TV would educate its viewers on how to prevent and cure disease with proper nutrition." Srdjan spoke with the optimism of a young, healthy man, with a clear picture in front of him.

Becket, Saturday, October 1, 1988

Another exciting day! I am in the kitchen with Bosko and Masao. I am the chef! Not even fifteen minutes had passed since we began cooking before I had a bad accident; I cut my index finger all the way to the bone. Fortunately, nobody noticed. I stormed down to the cellar where miso was stored and put miso on my finger, trying to fix it. The pain was unbearable! I was jumping around in circles and screaming at the top of my lungs. Fortunately the cellar had a thick, wooden door so nobody could hear me. It seemed as if the pain would never stop. Miso bit into my flesh but it cured the wound fast. The enzymes and the Vitamin B-12 helped it heal in two days.

Since nature healed my cancer I can stand pain more easily. I simply disregard the physical discharge, trying to connect with something beautiful in my imaginary world.

Becket, October 2, 1988

A new cloudy day dawned. The fog wrapped up the luxurious trees lining the slopes of the Berkshire mountains. This is the first morning we got up at 7 o'clock. It's probably because we are all so cosy and together. Srdjan has already started DO-IN in the library. Bosko, Yelena and I went on packing Srdjan's things without conversation. The atmosphere was strained. Then we had lunch together. We all chewed much longer than usual, wishing this afternoon would never end.

Yelena was the first to voice her feelings, "Mommy, I have a very restless butterfly under my chest bone. Whenever I think that Bata (the endearing name she calls her brother) has to go back to Boston, this butterfly in my chest goes crazy. I feel as if it's going to break through my chest."

Neither Bosko's nor my butterfly felt any better.

Our dear friend Masao understood our inner turmoil better than anyone. Somehow I felt he wanted to ease the pain of our family's separation. He appeared at our door with a warm smile on his face and a lunch box in his hand, addressing Srdjan.

"Jimi, (this is what everyone at the Kushi Institute called Srdjan), this will do you good if you get hungry on your way to Boston! There are also two cookies there, for a sweet trip."

I was more than touched by his gesture and I felt sudden warmth in my heart. Our friends here sympathize with us. They are part of our family now.

Srdjan left. We hoped he'd be back soon when he had no classes. There were mountains of joy ahead of us. The kind that energizes every day and makes life meaningful, full of color. Srdjan called back at seven o'clock, saying he'd arrived safely.

Rain started around eight. Fall arrived, bringing with it an easel of warm colors. In Massachusetts, fall is a most talented painter, author of the school of realism.

Becket, October 3, 1988

Today is cloudy and quite chilly. I cooked with Mrs. Kushi. Everything was flawless. I was personally happy with my work. So was my teacher.

She told an interesting story about a visit to Japan. She was served a cup of tea sweetened with plain white sugar which she hadn't eaten for some time. Not being aware of it, she sipped the tea. Instantly she got stomach cramps. A plaster made of tofu and greens relieved the pain quickly. We heard with astonishment that none of their five already grown-up children had ever seen a doctor. But they never ignore Western medicine. Just the opposite — their main teaching, their dream, is that traditional and modern medicine cooperate for the benefit of humanity.

Each encounter with my teachers brought a new discovery in the world of natural healing. Natural food is powerful medicine. Macrobiotics is the ultimate prevention in our struggle to stay healthy.

Days fly by in this earthly paradise. Nature's in ecstasy! The colorful hillsides of the Berkshire mountains are all in purple, violet, orange, yellow, brown and Tarner's (the artist) green hues. *"Is the universe having a party?!"*

Becket, October 15, 1988

It is my 46th birthday today. This is exactly one year and eight months from the date I was told that I was terminally ill, with two months to live. It's a sunny, warm Saturday. Our room is warm with love and contentment. If only Srdjan were here! Bosko and Yelena are asleep. I'm outside doing DO-IN exercises which strengthen inner organs. I feel my energy triple. Strength returns bringing inner peace and well being. Birds are singing in the trees. The sun is a shining crown in the sky. How is it possible to possess this much happiness? I possess no material riches, yet I am the richest person in the world. I have it all!

Returning to our room, Bosko and Yelena greeted me with a *"Happy Birthday"* song. I cried tears of happiness. What is Srdjan doing now I wondered. My unspoken question was answered. His telephone call awakened me from my dream. He wished me a happy birthday. He was O.K.

It's twenty past ten. Brunch is still not ready. Why so late this morning? The dining room table is covered with a tablecloth. What festivity is going on here, I ponder. Perhaps something in Mrs. Kushi's honor. She was in the kitchen with Masao and others. I peeped in. They were busy making Ohagi balls, prepared with sweet rice, chickpea powder, sesame seeds, azuki beans, lentils, squash and toasted walnuts. Extremely time consuming to prepare. Ahh, my favorite dessert! Nobody told me what was going on. "Brunch is served." What's that commotion in the kitchen?

Suddenly, Masao, Lily and Mariko appeared at the door singing: "Happy Birthday to you... dear Mina!"

I was caught by surprise. Tears streamed from my eyes.

"My dear friends! Thank you so much for everything! My happiness is complete. I will always remember this day!"

The celebration continued at "Ginga," a macrobiotic restaurant in Stockbridge. Bosko worked there part-time. Warmed by sake, we made tender love that night. I'm healthy and fulfilled. Now I know I'm alive! I know I'm going to live a long life!

Becket, November 4, 1988

After lunch, Bosko, Yelena, Hildegard (our new friend from Germany) and I went to Boston to be present at Srdjan's graduation ceremony. Luchi, our dear Spanish friend, told us that we could sleep in her family room at no charge. The Kushi Institute gave us a car to get to Boston. We were in heaven. We arrived at six-thirty right before dinner. Srdjan was thrilled to see us. We received many heartfelt greetings. They had heard about the Dobic family who had literally invaded the Kushi Institute.

After dinner Mr. and Mrs. Kushi made their appearance, accompanied by guests from Japan, the representatives of Mitoku Company, an international macrobiotic wholesale company. Mr. Kushi introduced Bosko as his friend from Yugoslavia.

Our happiest moment! Srdjan's name was announced as the youngest graduate ever of the Kushi Institute.

I have made it! I have lived to see my son graduate. This institute of macrobiotic learning equipped him with knowledge and skills sufficient to live a joyous and balanced life.

Attending Becket was like being at Harvard or Yale. The Dobics graduated as a family. Archimedes must have felt like this when he made the profound statement: *"Give me but one firm spot on which to stand and I will move the earth."*

Boston, November 30, 1988

Today we're in Boston. Our favorite U.S. city. We had driven Vera and Kuki, Yugoslavs from Zagreb, to the airport. Vera had lung cancer. Kuki was her constant shadow. He was so much in love with her. She was unwilling to accept a life philosophy different from her own. Kuki absorbed all possible knowledge during the week's workshop at Becket. His attempts to open a new door for her proved futile. He asked us for help but we had no success either.

"I cannot eat seeds and algae! I am a big woman! I have to get energy from meat. I can't eat a rabbit and bird diet! If you can eat it, Kuki, you are welcome. But then you are welcome to prepare it all yourself," she repeated.

We wished them well and waved our good-byes. Kuki called two months later. Vera had died.

From the airport we returned to Kushi House. Ate dinner with Yelena and Srdjan. Met two new friends, Zika, a Yugoslav, and his Japanese girl friend. Then attended the Kushi Institute Halloween party. Mariko made Yelena a great ghost costume. Srdjan dressed as an American tourist. Bosko, as a wealthy farmer from Dallas, (straight from a Soap Opera) and I was a Gypsy. We danced and sang. That was the most fun I had since my illness. We partied till after midnight. Time flew by too fast. I wanted this moment to last but we had to leave.

Next day we bought Srdjan a sweater, shirt and jeans. He was overjoyed. Everyone thought he was adorable. Bosko and I beamed with pride. I feel the power of their love deep in my soul. *Oh, my God, how much I love them!* Their love is my medicine.

"Smile, Mina, smile, even if you feel like crying," I told myself.

Becket, January, 1989

For me, "Introduction to Oriental Diagnosis," was the most interesting Level I class. Accurate diagnosis is the key factor in treating illness. A clear understanding of symptoms readily reveals the cause. An accurate diagnosis ensures correct healing recommendations. Oriental diagnosis requires neither expensive equipment nor elaborate technology. Your eyes, ears, nose, touch and intuition are the only tools employed. Of course, the sharper your instruments are honed, the more accurate your diagnosis will be.

The medicine of China, Japan and other Far Eastern countries is among the oldest in the world. This medicine teaches us a great deal that can be put into practice today. The basic philosophy of Oriental medicine is the complementary opposite of the kind of medicine currently practised in the West. Western medicine, with its emphasis on the treatment of symptoms by drugs and surgery, is increasingly powerless to cope with the rising tide of degenerative illness that now threatens to engulf the industrialized world. Clearly, we need to supplement our mainly symptomatic medicine with a medicine that is preventive in direction and humane and economical in application. Oriental medicine can contribute greatly to filling this need. Traditionally, this holistic diagnosis was used not only to study individuals but to analyze society as a whole.

They singled me out and used me as a model in class. Pointing to my chin, they said my main problem was with my reproductive organs. They were right on! And they had never seen my previous diagnosis. My teacher asked a pretty girl with sexy lips, her lower lip especially enlarged, to come forward. He pinpointed her major problem — constipation. And, again, he was right. Another student he observed had a large pimple on the tip of his swollen nose. The diagnosis was a weak heart, a heart murmur. The student admitted aloud that was correct.

Today, I learned that it is true that "Your Face Never Lies" [title of a book authored by Michio Kushi] because it is the mirror of your health. How fascinating! Illness can be recognized by skin color. Redness around the mouth indicates hypoglycemia and disorder in digestive system. Yellow color indicates pancreas, liver and gall bladder are in trouble. A greenish cast to the skin is seen in people developing a degenerative disease.

Wrinkles and lines on the face and body reveal tightness in corresponding organs. For example, there is meaning in the most common lines that develop on the face. Vertical lines between the eyebrows indicate liver condition. The deeper the lines, the more serious the problem.

This class had a profound effect on me. It was then I knew I would become a macrobiotic teacher and counselor, sharing these gems of knowledge with humanity. The methods of oriental diagnosis played a prominent role in all three levels I studied. Western medicine, the youngest healing art, identifies a disease by observation of its symptoms. Oriental medicine, the oldest traditional one, uses physiognomy as its principal tool — the art of judging a person "from the features of the face or the form and lineaments of the body generally." The Oriental diagnostician foresees the development of sickness before specific symptoms become apparent. We were trained to recognize and treat, but perhaps even more important, to *prevent* illness. Prevention is the most challenging, because with it comes the weighty responsibility of taking charge of one's own health.

That same day I bought Mr. Kushi's book, *How to See Your Health: Book of Oriental Diagnosis.* For the words I didn't know, I chased Yelena and Bosko around and asked for help. My teacher Michio Kushi told us how he had taught himself the art of diagnosis. He would take a day, go to the subway and study "noses" all day long. Next day he would only look at "eyes." Another day, only "lips." This is how he learned the finest distinctions and nuances between the hundreds of different noses, eyes and lips and other parts of the human body. By keen observation he discovered the overall health condition of society at large.

Becket, August 16, 1990

Today I graduated as a macrobiotic teacher! My exam reminds me and humbles me. It's been a long time since I played the role of the professor examining my students. Today, I stood on the other side. Not with stage fright, rather with honor. I wanted my teachers to be proud of their student. And they were! Because of my limited English, I had an oral exam. Srdjan stood by in case I needed an interpreter. I passed the oral exam smoothly and effortlessly.

Later this afternoon, I had the second phase of the exam, the cooking presentation. I chose "Medicinal Cooking for Lymphoma Cancer." It consisted of pressure-cooked short grain brown rice with millet, miso soup with daikon and tops, pan-fried (no oil) mochi (sweet pounded rice) filled with one teaspoon of grated daikon (a long white Japanese radish), seasoned with a few drops of soy sauce and ginger juice, wrapped with toasted Nori seaweed; hiziki seaweed dish with onion, carrots and lotus root; azuki beans with kombu seaweed and butternut squash; steamed collard greens with umeboshi plum (aged many years and pickled in salt) dressing. After cooking for two-and-a-half peaceful hours, I received a high grade and accomplished another goal. We were ready to return to our country and teach this New Way of Life.

That evening, we raised our sails. Announcing to the world our readiness for the next adventure.

Becket, August 26, 1990

The library in our dormitory was transformed into a disco. Sweaty bodies crowded inside swaying to rock and roll as it bounced off the walls. The Dobics are leaving and this is their farewell party. Everyone near and dear to us came to say their good-byes.

Thank God we rented a Budget van. We have enough room for all our presents. Tons of seaweed, miso, shiso leaves, tekka, kuzu, azuki and black soybeans, umeboshi plums and other very expensive macrobiotic food. Our friends knew that we could never get this in Yugoslavia.

Now the question arose: should we go home immediately or accept the invitation of our new friends in California to visit there awhile and then fly home. The vote came in: Srdjan and I wanted to see California, Bosko wanted to get home as quickly as possible, and Yelena was too young to vote. Farewell, Becket.

Chapter 11

California Dream

The next morning, with food enough for a month, cases of spring water, a compass, a map, an *International Macrobiotic Directory,* eight suitcases, two futons, two gas burners, a few pots and pans, a couple of disposable cameras, and a few dollars in our pocket — in short all our worldly belongings — we started our cross-country tour headed for the West Coast. The Berkshire Mountain "hillbillies" were ready to roll. Watch out world, here we come!

We were on the road for a month. We slept on futons in our rental van in parking lots at the best hotels. What a sight we made. The old folks in the back, preparing lunch to be served in our "private castle" at the next rest area stop. Kids in front. Srdjan driving at the same speed as the rock music blasting from the radio. Yelena knew all the words to the songs. They sang together at the top of their lungs.

The asphalt, hot enough to toast bread, unrolled beneath us, carrying us blissfully along from one state to another. As picturesque scenes of nature unfolded, we pulled to the side of the road for a better view. We were awestruck by the natural beauty of this vast country. Our eyes rushed over the ribbon of hillsides sprinkled alternately with brick homes and wood frame houses, vast plains, fascinating rock formations and inviting clusters of orange trees. The landscape peaked like a mountain dressed in her Sunday best, dotted with bushes, bursting with colorful trees yielding their petals of pink, filling the air with intoxicating perfume. On the far horizon we glimpsed a snow-tipped mountain. An occasional hill sloped gently from the sky. Ever so many tiny lakes were shaped like raindrops, colored heartbreak green. Each gentle whisper of nature, its sights and wonders, stole our breath away. Nature doesn't belong to anyone… but to everyone. Only selfishness and greed put borders on nature seeking to divide humanity. Wouldn't it be great to live like the birds who don't need passports?

With each new scenic discovery we shouted, "This should be the new wonder of the world." Travel is a life-enriching experience. It makes us wealthy, abundantly so. True riches come from a deep appreciation for nature's wondrous artistry and phenomena which remind us how small and arrogant we are. And how truly humble we should be.

I suggest we establish a National Holiday — *Return to Nature Day* — to celebrate the miracle of creation. It's been said, miracles are not contrary to nature but only contrary to what we know about nature. One day of each year, couldn't everyone choose one of nature's special creations: Yosemite, Sequoia, Sedona, the Rocky Mountains, Joshua Tree Park, Monument Valley, the Grand Canyon, Niagara Falls, or another untouched magical place anywhere in the world and peacefully gather as one family to cherish our universal heritage.

"Americans are so lucky," our kids repeated countless times. "Look at this country. All the seasons, different climates, are here for the taking. We don't want to go back to Yugoslavia. There's nothing as beautiful there."

Bosko's homesick voice betrayed his disappointment. He delivered his monologue, "What are you talking about? Your friends, your relatives are all there. You were born there. We have everything there. Our country is very beautiful."

"But it's nothing like this and we are very poor." They refused to give up their lament.

"Let's not spoil these beautiful moments. Enjoy the present," I said, trying to diffuse the tension.

They resumed their singing and entertainment program. As we rolled into Texas, Srdjan began his show. He imitated his favorite personalities. One by one we were visited by Al Pacino, Jerry Lewis, Joe Pesci, Humphrey Bogart and a few Yugoslav comedians for good measure. We laughed so hard we were swimming in our tears. Considering the length of time we had been traveling, we marveled at our storehouse of untapped reserves of energy. Nobody slept during the day. How could we? We were having too much fun. What a shift this was! We had just left a quiet, almost sacred place. Suddenly we found ourselves in this wide open, free and easy, aimless adventure, balancing ourselves with new found abandon.

One by one, a pearl string of nature's elegant beauties, each one different, renewed our excitement with each new discovery. We loved every place we visited. We all fell in love with Arizona. Santa Fe, New Mexico was one of our favorite places. Just two hours before arriving in Colorado Springs, the white bride of the mountains, our van's air conditioner died. We drenched ourselves with spring water. Pouring bottle after bottle over our heads in an attempt to forget the sizzling 105 degree temperature.

In each state along the way, we stopped to visit macrobiotic friends whom we had met while at the Kushi Institute. We felt as if we were members of a huge family. They welcomed us warmly, gave us the run of the house and stuffed our bags with food for our trip. That was a big relief. We didn't have to cook every day. The kids were even happier. They didn't have to wash dishes.

Bosko was out-numbered two to one. Our destination was to be sunny California, the state with the highest taxes and fewest jobs. How brave we were with only a couple of dollars left. Never could we have imagined what was about to happen. And happen it did.

After two weeks of sightseeing in California, we had planned to return home. But this was not to be. CNN broke the news: Yugoslavia was engaged in Civil War! Silence, tears, fear and sorrow, all rushed in. Repeated phone calls weren't getting through. We were in shock. What were they fighting for? Another page turned! It seemed our life must begin over again!

Our new homestead: one 300 square foot room in a friend's home. We played new roles: housekeeper, cook, butler, driver, and baby-sitter in exchange for our room. Thanks be to God we had a lot of expensive food already. After being at Becket, honored and appreciated, this existence was degrading. Our closeness and mutual love and our new life philosophy enabled us to survive. In those most difficult moments, I drew strength from the knowledge that I had survived cancer. We could survive this, too. And we did.

Two months later, we found a place of our own in Costa Mesa, California. It was close to a health food store, which was important to us because we had no car. It only took us a few days to settle in. Srdjan started Orange County College. Yelena enrolled in Mariner's Elementary School. Bosko got his first housekeeping job for a wealthy Newport Beach doctor. He divided his time between chasing after her most prized possession, her dog, and... ironing ladies' underwear! Something he'd never done before and prays he will never have to do again. Poor Bosko! He felt humiliated. He didn't care if there was a war. He wanted to leave immediately. He was even willing to walk there if he had to. Anything is better than this, he thought.

I started teaching cooking classes and preparing macrobiotic meals for take-out. Life was merciful but not for Bosko. Fortunately, by the second month, he got a good job at the hospital. That same week, we bought our first car at a garage sale for $200 cash and three bikes. Good buys! We were elated!

Shortly thereafter I became known as a macrobiotic leader. Word spread about the benefits of implementing balance in one's life. An educational program was organized by Mother's Market and Kitchen, the nearby health food store. I started giving lectures regularly. In a year-and-a-half, their macrobiotic section and sales expanded three times. This resulted from their accepting my recommendations to enlarge their selection of macrobiotic products and carrying a wider variety of organic food.

Our life took on a new direction. I started receiving phone calls nationally and internationally. People wanted to do work-study programs with me. I was thrilled that so many of them were young people, highly educated, who valued a better quality of life. One and all, they were welcome in our home. They came from Europe, Australia, South America, and Africa. Our guests adopted us as part of their families. For all of them, the door of our home was always open. We meant that literally. They had a key to our home and we never changed the locks!

With new friends from all over the world, Srdjan and Yelena felt like citizens of the world. They used their knowledge and experience with macrobiotics to help their friends. Many of them became healthier and happier, giving up meat, dairy and sugar.

We made many new friends in Costa Mesa and Newport Beach. To me, helping others was not about getting rich at their expense. Many people who came to me couldn't afford to pay but I never turned them away. Fortunately, there were enough who could afford it. I used a portion of that money to purchase food and books for those who didn't have money.

As our friends grew in number and our kids got older, our two-bedroom apartment became too crowded. We moved to larger quarters, still in the same neighborhood. It didn't take long to move because we didn't have much furniture. While we were still unpacking, the phone rang. It was Gwen Staats inquiring whether we would be home that afternoon. She asked Bosko to come over right away. A few hours later, our new apartment was decorated with beautiful antique furniture, including a piano... compliments of our dear friends, the Staats family!

Whenever Bosko had bouts of homesickness, I would try to encourage him:

"Home is in your heart. It doesn't matter where you live, if you're happy. You couldn't be happy living in an atmosphere of hate, dealing with prejudice, in a homeland torn apart by war."

"Yes, you are right," the lines on his forehead stretching like an accordion, the light returning to his eyes.

In the midst of all this, a sad day arrived. We had lived in California three years when we got the news. My father, my hero, died of a broken heart in the tender arms of his loving son. He had been watching the news on TV soon after civil war had spread to Bosnia. Tired of all the human stupidity, the old, proud hero deserted the world of consciousness, choosing peace, the holy peace.

The news came as Srdjan was cutting his cake celebrating his twenty-first birthday. The phone rang. My brother spoke in a breathless voice, "I don't know what to say first — Happy Birthday, Srdjan, or your Grandpa just left us forever." It was May 25th 1993. Day of Youth, a national celebration and the birthday of ex-President Tito. I firmly believe that father chose that day to die as his final act of defiance. By so doing, he overtly and boldly underlined a part of corrupt history with his own honorable life.

That day I marked the calendar with the words, "Another root of my life dried up." Now I had lost both parents. I was prevented from being there to receive my last blessing because of bureaucratic paperwork. Life's scars are full of pain. It takes a long time to heal.

Flashback!

The year is 1953. A shy, quiet, studious, petite girl dares to dream big. All the lights in the house are off. One light secretly

shines under mountains of heavy blankets over her bed. Her dou-
bled-up body hides the latest issue of "Film Magazine." She
adroitly stole it from her aunt's nightstand soon after she left with
her boyfriend. Gregory Peck and Audrey Hepburn are together
in Roman Holiday. And she is there, too! The light flickers in her
gentle hand. When the light is on, she's captivated reading about
the "stars." When she turns the light off, she sees herself as her
favorite female star. She is Audrey Hepburn in Roman Holiday
with Gregory Peck. If her mother knew what was going on under
her blanket, a punishment worse than death would be imposed
upon her: no more movie-going for a year. She would disappear
inside herself with suffering, being deprived of her most cherished
dream… to be in Hollywood.

After all those years, that little girl is now living her dream! She came not
to become an actor, or to seek stardom. No trumpets announced her arrival.
But rather, she quietly stole on the scene committing herself to instilling hope
and promise in the lives of those who had none. She worked tirelessly and
sincerely took a personal interest in making sure that other people's dreams
came true.

Traveling in California, I "discovered" Hollywood first. I didn't know it at
the time but I had a special mission to minister to those searching for hope, a
search I had completed eleven years earlier. Practically speaking, I learned the
meaning of the maxim: "We are not born into this world to do everything but
to do something."

My fee for students and children has always been "no charge." That's my
contribution to a better world. The little something I gave came from the
depths of my being. I gave wholeheartedly. I held nothing back. And an
amazing thing happened!

I was welcomed within the Hollywood circle as a person highly
recognized in her field. My clients include many Hollywood producers,
directors, actors, and other well-known celebrities.

Srdjan arrived in Hollywood second. He is not yet living his dream. He
wants to be a movie director and is working hard toward that goal. Presently
he is working on a script and hopes to exert a positive influence on human
lives.

My daughter, Yelena, an outstanding student in her junior year, hopes to follow him with her dream to be an entertainment attorney. "When I get tired of dealing with law, I may become a Hollywood producer and work with my brother. And then we'll complete Mom's dream by giving her a role in Srdjan's movie."

My precious husband of 27 years still loves me. He gently, constantly wraps the children and me with his love and joyful surprises. He has devoted his life to us and our dream of One Peaceful World.

The year is 1996. Only in America could we play the lead roles in this fairytale story. Two guardian angels spun the Wheel of Fortune for the Dobics, setting our roots firmly in American soil. Our dearest friends, Phyllis Mueller and Glenn Warren, entrepreneurs and owners of a very successful multi-million dollar international business, have been more than just our family's financial pillars of support for the last two years. Their generosity extends to countless others as well. Phyllis and Glenn are also the "Godfathers" of this book. In the Fall of 1996, they presented us with the keys to our new home, swimming pool and all, and moved us into it!

Life is happiest for them when they are making other people happy. Money for them is not the issue. Making a difference in people's lives is. That which we treasure most about these endearing friends is the loving relationship we share. We've fashioned a secret pocket, sewn close to our hearts, that overflows with the love they have given us. We shall keep it there always, cherishing their friendship in a very special way.

Continually helping countless people with cancer, I observed a common thread emerging. They accepted the diet and lifestyle changes and progressed but something was missing. They felt they were alone. That no one understood what they were going through. In the majority of cases, their families weren't able to give the support they sorely needed.

Two of my former clients, cancer survivors, now among my dearest friends, gave birth to the idea of establishing a weekly Macrobiotic Support Group. One of them opened her home for the weekly gathering. For a year-and-a-half, I was privileged to lecture and support them on a weekly basis. Every Monday we made the hour-long trip to Hollywood Hills. At my suggestion they invited other teachers, who came from across the country and other continents. From that small beginning five years ago, this group has continued to grow and become well known.

I have personally experienced what Oriental philosophy teaches those who practice the macrobiotic way of life: "You give unconditionally, you receive unconditionally. When you balance correctly, eat well, exercise, care about others, live in harmony with nature, have gratitude and appreciation for whatever happens, everything will come to you — *because you create your own destiny.*"

Chapter 12

Healing Stories

1. A Blessed Event
by Alex Downs and Tammy ann Casper

Tammy ann and I are both professionals in the entertainment industry. We have always tried to eat healthy food prepared at home. We thought that giving up red meat and eating a modified-vegetarian diet that included chicken a few times a week would be healthy and wise. For our generation this seemed to be "the cure" to bad living. Yet we didn't feel revitalized by our lifestyle even though we exercise regularly. A chance meeting with Nadine Barner, a macrobiotic cook and angel, sent us on a quest that would begin with quinoa, a strange "queen's grain" and would include foods that we had never eaten before in our lives and others that we just didn't know to eat regularly or in certain quantities.

There is a strange unmasking that takes place with Mina, and with your relationship to food, when you begin this quest. Quite literally Mina was able to read our faces, our skin, our smiles and knew what ailed us. At this time Tammy ann and I had also decided that we wanted to have a child and Tammy ann was dedicated to cleansing her body and her mind to prepare herself for this physical and emotional transition. With that in mind, Mina put us on a six week macrobiotic cleansing diet that helped to educate us on the energy and harmony available through the principles of macrobiotic eating.

Though it took some getting used to (it takes will to change old habits), we turned our philosophy and practice of eating food upside down and discarded everything in our kitchen that was not organic or that contained preservatives, sugar or hydrogenated oils. In their place we included organic grains of all types, fresh organic produce, beans, seeds, soy, sea vegetables, noodles, things we had never tried that left us feeling rejuvenated.

Tammy ann's pregnancy under macrobiotics was amazing. After being together for 15 years and not trying to get pregnant, we conceived our child the first week we tried, where as friends of ours struggled month after month spending thousands of dollars pumping fertility drugs into their system. Tammy ann ultimately gained a healthful 30 pounds and exercised throughout her pregnancy while the baby got the most incredible foundation of nutrition imaginable. Another amazing by-product of macrobiotics seemed to be that Tammy ann never experienced any morning sickness and had abundant energy throughout the day.

When the baby was born we knew someone special had joined our family. From the very first moment of her new life little Liberty Rae was filled with alert, wide-eyed wonder. She looked upon her Momi and Popi and this incredible new world she was born into with probing, soulful interest. Her clear complexion and serene disposition astound us every day and we attribute this to our love, the healthy foundation Tammy ann gave her and the macrobiotic-produced breast milk that she eats exclusively.

Incredibly, at three months of age, we ask her where our nose, eyes and mouth are and she touches them to show her understanding. She has the most incredible smile and radiant laugh and loves to stand on her own two feet as she holds our hands for balance. *Balance.* That is ultimately the principle that makes so much sense about macrobiotics. Getting your body into balance so that it can function the way God intended in a synchronous dance with the abundance that nature provides season to season.

For us this has been a doorway into a new way of life that has spiritually and physically revitalized us. We look years younger, our clarity of thought, our complexions, our soul, Tammy ann's pregnancy, our child have all benefited from this education. What particularly impressed us was the principle that live food sustains the soul in ways that change your spirit because it feeds you life. When we have eaten dead food we have felt deadened, as if the rot of this food were slowing us down and saddening our spirit. Living in harmony with the earth in macrobiotic balance changed us on a cellular level and we are so thankful to Nadine and Mina for helping us make this transformation. A renaissance of the mind, body and soul takes place when you follow this path. Start walkin'.

2. *They Sent Him Home to Die*

Peter, four-year-old son of Anna and Adam, is terminally ill with cancer of the urinary tract. Their search for hope for their son has brought them to me. Even a casual glance tells you he has suffered a lot. His little head is bald. His cute round face is greenish-gray. There are dark circles under his chestnut brown eyes, devoid of light, as if they belong to an old man. His thin, colorless lips, hiding under his button nose, have lost their joy of smiling. He can't eat because his mouth is sore, full of painful canker sores. His tiny body is so skinny it's hard to find it under his baggy clothing.

I ask myself, how could any therapy be really good when it damages the body so unmercifully? How could such aggressive treatment help an already weak immune system in the process of recovery? Here's a child whose life is over before it barely gets started. He isn't just wasting away; his entire being, physically, emotionally and spiritually, is being destroyed. It is obvious that his life is dimming. His doctors told them that there is nothing more they can do for Peter so they sent him home to die.

Anna is a 25-year-old attractive woman with pleasing proportions, but her oval face displays a cold, painful, involuntary cramp-like expression. Her sapphire eyes no longer sparkle. They appear puffy and lined with red. As she finds the most comfortable position on the sofa, she unconsciously uses her long, slender fingers to comb through her hair. The sunlight catches the brilliance of her diamond as she struggles nervously to untangle the hair that winds around her expensive ring. Even the costly thick, gold chain that adorns her sculptured neck cannot restore life to her face. Yet in spite of her pain, she still radiates a strong spirit from within. This same strong spirit has been genetically inherited by Peter.

Adam is blond and very tall, obviously a body-builder. His hands move nervously. His face is ruddy and when he talks, his utterances are angry and judgmental.

His young parents have reached an impasse regarding Peter's healing. Anna wants to use the macrobiotic approach while Adam doesn't believe in macrobiotics. Adam is of the opinion that it's cruel to give his son false hope because he doesn't believe food causes illness, let alone cure it. (This belief is almost universally shared by health professionals and the science community.) Adam was close to yelling at Anna. "I don't want my son to starve to death eating bird food, grains, beans, and seaweed. He'll die even sooner without meat. Not only that, but who's going to cook that 'microbiotic' food when the only thing you cook is coffee?!"

Within this family exists a horrendous conflict. Anna is a strict vegetarian. Adam is a meat-eater. He also drinks heavily. Their son Peter is inclined to favor his father's diet. So the real conflict is not about Peter's lifestyle but about whose ego is to be satisfied. Anna is ready to use food as medicine for her son's healing. But Adam thinks it's too much pressure to deprive Peter of the food he likes, especially now that cancer has taken over his life.

How sad it is to see this family, which is really no family at all but a mere pretense. At a time when Peter's life is being measured in seconds, he becomes the victim of his parent's blind selfishness. That negative energy conceals the real issue: What preserves and nourishes human life? So I'm watching them and wondering, "Where is the love, unconditional/unselfish love?" Then as I look at Peter, I sense he has made a decision to leave his parents — to die. His little face has darkened as his head has dropped and he looks to me like an old man, exhausted with life, who has decided his life is over.

"Excuse me," I say. "Please help me to understand the purpose of your visit. Your child's destiny is in your hands. If you continue to argue, I don't see any solution." I said this in an attempt to move the conversation along.

"Adam," Anna confronted him. "We came here hoping to find a way to help our child. Let's allow Mina to introduce this diet to us."

"Do you know what macrobiotics is about?" I ask. "Do you know what that word means?"

They silently shook their heads from side to side. Anna added, "I did some reading but I don't know enough. I'm willing to learn."

I explained to them that macrobiotics essentially means "large life" and the diet is based on a common-sense approach using natural, whole grains and organic vegetables. "In your son's case," I said, "since he's only four years old, you both must assume that responsibility for him. Didn't you already tell me that the doctors didn't help him?"

Anna interrupts, and turning toward her husband begins to speak, "Yes. We went to the doctors. We allowed them to do whatever they said had to be done, never questioning any treatment they prescribed. They proposed a special study program. Over the past two years, Peter was treated with radiation and chemotherapy. Nothing worked. Now we're looking for another approach. That's why we're here. Peter hasn't even tried macrobiotics. We came to you to learn about it. Adam, you immediately show that you discount the value of this alternative approach. But what about Mina? She is a cancer survivor. Will you discount her so quickly, too?"

She continued. "I've read a lot of books and I've been trying to share everything I've learned with you. You refuse to read or listen to anything. In fact, those books are still sitting unopened on the nightstand next to your bed." Adam looked down and remained silent.

Observing them was like watching two children on a seesaw in rapid motion, afraid any minute that one would fall off and Peter will be the one feeling the most pain. I already felt his pain and hopelessness and, unconsciously, moved from my chair to the floor. At that moment, Peter accepted my silent invitation to sit on my lap.

Looking into his sad eyes, I said to him, "I guess you don't like it when your parents are talking this way."

He shook his little head from side to side. "No."

"What else don't you like?"

"I don't like when people shoot the birds and I don't like when I have to stop playing with my friends when I feel pain."

"What do you do when you have pain?" I saw his lips twitch.

"Me and my mom pray to Jesus and sometimes I have to go to the hospital, lose my hair and watch those stupid cartoons."

"Do you watch cartoons at home?"

"Yes."

"Are they stupid?"

"No."

"Why do you say that hospital cartoons are stupid?"

"Because they *are* stupid and the hospital is stupid and all those machines in my room are stupid and the food is yukkie," he insisted.

"You are not going to go there again!" I promised him. He dove deeper into my lap and held on tight.

"I don't want to."

I hugged him tightly and said, "Let's pray together that you don't have to go there." He rested his cold, petite hands in my arms and whispered with me, "Dear Jesus, please don't ever let Peter have to watch cartoons in the hospital and don't let him have those machines attached to him, not even in his dreams. Stop all the pain in Peter's body with pure and healthy food. Let him play and play and play with his friends until he gets tired playing. Thank you, Jesus." And I heard a deep sigh as he whispered "Amen." Then I broke the silence. "Peter, shall we ask your mom and dad to join us on the floor?"

Teary eyed, he said, "If they want."

Gladly they joined us, moving closer to their son and gathering him into their warm embrace. This was just what was needed to turn the situation around.

The room became intensely hot. I wanted to leave so their love could take my place. For a second I felt like an intruder and that I should absent myself, for this was their moment. It belonged to them alone.

Adam was the first to say, "Let's hear what Mina has to say."

I introduced macrobiotics to them and designed a healing diet specific to Peter's needs. I also gave them a few names of people who recovered from the same illness using the macrobiotic way of healing. They left in peace.

For the first time in her life, Anna took charge and became the chief pharmacist in her "Pharmacy of Life" — her own kitchen. She spent hours and hours cooking meals, making medicine for her son and herself.

One day all three of us were cooking in the kitchen. We made Peter's favorite dish — French fries! He was busy eating them as fast as he could cook them saying "Yummy, yummy, yummy." He didn't notice that he was really making "turnip" French fries! I remember thinking how unusual this was: seeing a man (even a four-year-old boy) in the kitchen. In my country, people think it is degrading for a man to be in the kitchen, doing 'woman's work.'

Three months later, Peter's test revealed incredible improvement. And after six months, he was cancer free! Unfortunately, his parents had already divorced but despite this Peter is today a happy and healthy child.

3. My Healing Journey
by Antoinette Ippolito, M.Ed.

I am 53 years old and conscious that time is precious. In 1996, within a few months, I experienced many life-wrenching changes: I had gotten married, been laid off from work, and moved into a new home. I kept wondering, "How is it that I have gone through so many changes without getting sick?" The answer came in the middle of January.

My period began again after an absence of two months. I was very happy to see it arrive. It continued for a week, then 10 days... then two weeks. At this point, Don and I went to the movies one Saturday night. When we got home and saw I was bleeding heavily, I panicked. "I'm scared," I said to him. "I'm still flowing and I feel like I'm fading away." Watching your vital essence pass from your body is a horrifying sight and I knew something was wrong.

Years ago, I had read a book called *Recalled by Life*, by Anthony Satillaro. It is the story of a medical doctor's battle with terminal prostate cancer and his eventual cure with macrobiotics.

I had studied macrobiotics years ago and had practised it for a while but not with any full commitment. But through my study of macrobiotics I had come to know an excellent macrobiotic diagnostician/advisor who lived near me. Her name was Mina Dobic and she has always been one of the people whom I am truly thankful to have in my life.

At the instance of having my period for two weeks, I called Mina and begged her for an appointment. My intuition told me that I might have fibroids, an affliction which my mother had, resulting in a partial hysterectomy. Mina agreed to see me that Monday.

When I arrived for my appointment, I was nearly hysterical. I was weak from blood loss, but was also – and probably just as debilitating – scared to death! Mina saw my state and we sat together for almost an hour-and-a-half. She asked me what I was eating and what was going on in my life both emotionally and spiritually. Part of my problem was that my marriage with Don had been, up to now, a strain on me.

I had also been eating badly. I knew better. But lately I had been consuming sweets, meat, coffee, wine – all of which I knew were wrong. The eating was a feeble attempt to alleviate stress and to get some pleasure in my life.

Mina checked my pulses, looked at my face, my hands, assessed the puffiness and swelling, the whites of my eyes, my overall weight gain. She said she believed I had fibroids and told me that they are not necessarily related to menstruation nor necessarily to mid-life, but are the result of excess accumulations in the body from years of stress and over-consumption of sugar, oil and animal products.

This, compounded by the numerous life changes I had recently experienced, had resulted in unwanted growths. She said they were a warning sign and that I had to make a radical change if I were to get well. She also suggested that she couldn't proceed further until I had a pelvic ultra scan to determine the size, number and location of them.

After our consultation, I went home with a copy of the standard macrobiotic diet, which included her specific recommendations and immediately went to the natural food store and began my shopping.

From the beginning of January, when I first saw Mina, to the end of January, I bled for a total of 23 days. Those last 10 days I was in hell. I was very frightened about the betrayal of my body but realized I had to bite the bullet and take care of myself. My saving grace was the support of my girl friends, to whom I told everything. They called me several times a day and allowed me to be as panicky as I wished, accepting me exactly the way I was.

I decided to begin macrobiotics because I felt it was the smartest thing I could do. It was tough for I had no help immediately at hand. I felt miserable, had lost weight, was pale and weak, terrified, and I had to do my own food shopping and food preparation. Mina suggested what to do and allowed me to call her several times with questions, which she patiently answered at each instance. But I had to take care of myself.

Wrestling with the fear was bad enough. Wrestling with my own mind and its resistance to this task, which at the time seemed insurmountable, was almost as bad. I sat at the kitchen counter, praying and saying aloud to myself, "You are capable. The bottom line is that no one can do it for you. You can do this. You have to do this."

Motivated by the fact that Mina would work with me only after a confirmation of her diagnosis, I called my doctor and demanded a referral for the ultra scan. I got the referral and somehow drove myself to the hospital to have the procedure done. While on the freeway, my hands were shaking on the steering wheel. I was a wreck and on the examining table, kept saying, "Do you see anything? What's there?" I know that I drove the technician crazy and was completely amazed when she said she saw nothing of significance.

I jumped off the table, ecstatic and called Mina to say they couldn't find anything. She paused for a few seconds and said, "Then you should be very happy."

About a week later, the doctor's office called me to say that there were indeed two fibroids but they were small. They therefore considered the ultra scan to be "normal." I called Don and told him, then telephoned Mina. She said, "You can shrink them. Let's get to work."

Realistically, 'combination medicine,' which blends East and West, may be the best bet. But I decided that at this juncture, I myself would make the essential lifestyle changes in an attempt to heal myself of all the negatives which I had allowed into my life, dietary and otherwise.

I then met my own resistance head on. I sometimes sat at the kitchen table at 3:30 in the morning, wondering where to start. I made food charts and wrote out every single item I was to eat daily, two times a week, three times, or weekly. I made a master shopping list. I literally dragged myself to the natural food store. I took the capsules Mina had suggested. I went for short walks. I ate well.

I watched reruns of "The Andy Griffith Show" to calm me down. I did deep breathing. I prayed to God. And the bleeding lessened. And by the end of January stopped.

I felt there had been a miracle in my life! And I had done it with my own hands, under my own steam. I got down on my hands and knees and thanked my Creator for inspiring me to do what I had to do.

Several months have passed. The symptoms are gone and the fibroids are reduced by half. My cholesterol reading, always high, is down by 112 points! But I still have work to do, all is not perfect. Like a total fool, I have strayed a few times from the alkaline, clean food that was prescribed. I have lost about 20 pounds but most of them were bloaty fat that was ugly to me. On good days, I feel as if I am floating, with high energy and a calm, centered feeling. On some days, when the food preparation seems overwhelming to me, I remind myself, at Mina's behest, that I am healing myself.

I have also streamlined my cooking process, so that it takes less time. I enjoy the food, which can be as delicious as any other but with less spices and no animal products. I mainly use fresh, organic vegetables, beans and bean products and whole grains. When I go out, I take my food with me, since I am still in the initial healing phase. Later, I may be able to eat simple foods, such as pasta, in restaurants. But I don't think I'll ever go back to the artificial, over-spiced fare which I had been eating all my life. It now tastes bizarre to me and seems synthetic and fake. I can no longer tolerate anything phony in my life, not even cheesecake.

To anyone who reads this, I would ask you to appraise your life and courageously do something while you can. And to realize that in the end, the power of love and helping yourself and others, is all there is. I would ask you to be good to yourself and practice this. Be kind to the fellow human being who may be seated next to you, who is trying to live the precious life she was given by God in the best way she knows how.

4. A Day in the Life of Mina

I started preparing meals for my family at 5 o'clock this morning. Now it's about noontime, another warm, sunny day in California. I'm relaxing in a lounge chair next to the pool in my back yard. The birds are composing their sonatas while I, their audience of one, am touched in a special way by their musical concert. I feel compelled to thank them for their performance. And as I talk to them, they respond by raising their voices in harmony. It's as if they are speaking a new language and I'm the only who understands it. I believe they know my mood and they come looking for me. They possess an uncanny ability to be there at the moment when I need them. The musical message they bring me makes me feel special. I am grateful yet overwhelmed by this phenomenon.

The rhythmic sound of the water as it flows from the Jacuzzi into the pool is the river of my childhood. It resonates through my body, gently delivering me into deep meditation. In these pleasant surroundings, I feel the knotted tightness uncoiling and the chapel of my soul being blessed. My mind is expanding with nature's vibrations. Again I renew my connection with the universe. The doorbell breaks this magical spell.

My daughter, Yelena, opens the door. Standing in the door frame is a young woman, my size, my age, wearing the same cramp-like expression on her face which I once wore. How well I know the meaning of that expression, I lived with it for so many years. There she was, the personification of the Mina I once was. It was like looking in the mirror and seeing myself. For one brief moment, it was frightening.

When she opened her heart and told her story, it was deja vu. As her story unfolded, she recounted her lifestyle: director of a TV sit-com, wholly devoted to her career, last one to leave the studio, loses track of time, forgets to eat, forgets to use the bathroom, weekends devoted to preparing for next week's program, no picnics, no vacation, no private life.

Scary, isn't it. She didn't know where to start. She didn't know how to stop. She knew she was on a treadmill and couldn't get off. She knew she couldn't take it any more. Chronic fatigue syndrome, recurring migraines, chronic allergies, digestive disorders, acute candida, PMS, all chipping away at her ability to concentrate, to function. Choking her! Years of medication had produced only temporary change and destructive side effects. Medications can only target symptoms, generate new causes.

Like most people, she wanted to know what caused her condition. I proceeded to explain relevant facts.

"Candida is an infection by a yeast-like fungus similar to parasites which lives in the body without any ill effects. It affects the moist skin areas of the body, oral mucous membranes, respiratory tract and vagina. As it increases in intensity, it can enter the blood stream, penetrate cell walls, inhabit different organs, even cross the blood-brain barrier."

The key to her cure was to avoid fermented foods, excepting umeboshi plum, which is used extensively for medicinal cooking. Candida thrives on a sugary climate. So it was important to avoid simple carbohydrates, such as pastries with yeast, fruits, any sweeteners and raw salt added to cooked food. Weak kidneys cannot maintain the proper amount of sodium in the bodily fluids.

In order to cure candida and build up the immune system, one must first strengthen the kidneys. She was advised to apply ginger compresses on her kidneys for 20 minutes twice a week. This compress improves blood circulation and brings needed oxygen to the kidneys, thereby strengthening them. Thirty minute salt baths twice a week were recommended. Even when a person knows that she should, it's hard to give up familiar foods. The spirit is strong but the body is weak.

Nancy confided in me, "On one occasion on the set, we were forced to stop shooting because I was too sick to continue. As it turned out, that was good because I met the person who told me about you. Her story is my story. She gave me your phone number."

Before we started her consultation, one by one, she took each prescription drug, all the vitamins, minerals and other supplements from her purse. "Where is your garbage can? I have been on this stuff for years and look what it's doing to me. I want to get rid of it once and for all," she said angrily.

This was her first introduction to macrobiotics, so I gave her a brief overview. Our world today is technologically powerful but it's out of balance. Disease, increased crime, high divorce rates, biogenetic engineering, are all evidence of rampant disorder that ultimately leads to human annihilation. The macrobiotic approach could be used to heal suffering and restore balance. Food is the only energy powerful enough to heal our physical, emotional and spiritual being.

Food can heal the world but you have to put macrobiotic tools into practice. Eat only organic food and work to see that food is organically grown; exercise; live in harmony with nature and the environment; be grateful for the gift of life; distribute joy and thankfulness to all of mankind.

This brief philosophical approach made sense to Nancy. Her comment was that she lived and worked in an ignorant and angry world. She was ready to change. When was the last time she walked in the daylight or after a meal? She couldn't remember. The only exercise she got was walking from the car to her front door, studio or restaurant. She understood that we are part of nature and we have to go back to nature. Everything we put in our body and on our body, should be natural and pure.

It took her awhile to accept the dietary changes. She stopped abusing her body with meat, dairy and sugar, but she had a hard time giving up fruit and pastry. Those were the hardest habits to break. She didn't like to cook but took care of that simply by hiring a macrobiotic cook. In two months her symptoms were gone. Even after recovering she decided to keep her cook. But now she selects her food from a "gourmet" macrobiotic menu.

As her condition improved, not only did the old symptoms vanish but her skin became satiny and wrinkles softened. She looked ten years younger. She became calm, her depression subsided and she was able to concentrate once again. As people complimented her, she told them her "secret." She shared her story with everyone who would listen. Many people benefitted and made changes in their lives as well. Once again, the maxim is true: "From one grain, ten thousand grains."

Nancy and I became good friends and expanded our relationship. There was no more counselor and client. There was only friend and friend. I lost count of how many times we cooked together, took walks together. She made a profound discovery, or at least it was to her. The birds had always been here. The birds had always been singing but she had never heard them. Attending their command performance was playful, like living in a never ending fairytale world. Adopting the macrobiotic way of life enabled her to discover the highest level of consciousness, the dynamics of infinite freedom and a quality of life that completes our health and internal happiness. Life is a symphony and we are the conductors.

5. A Story of Healing
by Jennifer E. Greene, Ph.D.

It is December 1988 and the holiday season is in full swing. I learned a few weeks ago that my husband was having an affair and now a biopsy has revealed that I have breast cancer. I cannot say that I am in shock, as many women are when this news is delivered. It is more surprising, not that cancer came but that it came so early. My mother was fifty-eight when hers began. I am forty-four.

My mother had a radical mastectomy with her first cancer and another ten years later with her second. She died ten years after that following several rounds of chemotherapy. The cancer had spread to her bones, her brain, her being. My "A-team" (as one of them liked to put it) of L.A. doctors decided a lumpectomy, radiation and tamoxifen were reasonable treatment. I know that something more is being called for, beyond medical treatment. I cannot buy my doctors' view that cancer is a meaningless tragedy. I know that something in the way I am living is causing it, something related to forty-four years of feeling powerless, as if I am not yet really living but always getting ready to live.

For many years, I have felt that my real self is near but that I am cut off from her. Only when I drink — as I did in great quantity between the ages of twenty and forty — do I have intimations of her spunk, her liveliness, her creativity.

I leave my job at the Motion Picture Association and start helping others use dance to break free of old, confining ways. Alone in my living room late one night I watch the film *Out of Africa*. As I watch Isak Dinesen lose everything that matters to her, I find the core of myself that is a survivor.

The shame lifts and briefly I feel freer that I can remember. Then I find a new lump. Because of a needle biopsy that wrongly characterizes the lump as benign, I leave it there from September 1991 until January of 1992, when a rising tumor marking blood test arouses my oncologist's suspicion. Once again I undergo a lumpectomy. This time my doctors strongly urge chemotherapy but I again opted for radiation. I still see my little lumps as local phenomena. Attacking the whole body with deadly chemicals strikes me as overkill.

I have not yet stopped to ask why my body is growing malignant lumps. What is in there that makes those lumps pop up? Then in July 1992, I am faced with a more difficult dilemma: the cancer has spread to my sternum. I no longer have the option of a tidy little surgery to remove it. With heart and lungs so close, neither is my old stand-by radiation advisable. It seems chemotherapy is my only choice. I have two treatments, a week apart, and then something happens I am still at odds to explain.

In September 1991, when I thought I was quite happily settled in a relationship that seemed both supportive and strong, I surprised myself by falling wildly in love with a man several years my junior. I do not know what to say about destiny or changing one's destiny. But it seems quite possible that had I stayed in that former relationship with a man who was a cancer survivor himself, yet had an ineradicable fear-based faith in Western medicine, I would not be here today. This new man has an understanding that there are ways to cleanse a body naturally, an idea which I, with my conventional medical thinking, regard dubiously.

Yet, as I look back now, something clearly had been set in motion and getting connected with Scott was preparation for what happened next. We visit a holistic M.D. who suggested macrobiotics as nutritional support for chemotherapy. On September 1st 1992, I meet with Mina. She tells me, among many other things, that clearing the cancer from my body will be a piece of cake. This is in striking contrast to my oncologist's view that chemotherapy will probably take care of this round but that there is a ninety percent chance it will recur.

By now I do not know what is moving me. Maybe it is Mina's inspiring encouragement. Maybe it is my oncologist's discouraging view. Maybe it is my significant other's report on every negative nuance of change resulting from two chemotherapy treatments. Maybe it is the sensation that my teeth are coming loose. Maybe it is all of the above and maybe none. Somewhere in me the decision is made, perhaps by a part of me that knows more than the I who usually makes decisions, to leave Western medicine and embark on a journey of macrobiotic healing.

Life on my macrobiotic regime is about getting simple. Scott and I learn the cooking together and our kitchen becomes our pharmacy. I scrub my body with hot ginger water morning and night to improve circulation and move stagnation. I go for long walks, getting out into nature at every opportunity. I sing happy songs. I wear pure cotton next to my skin. I avoid television with all the pollution it cranks out. I wear a cabbage plaster on the area over my sternum to pull the toxins out. Sometimes I feel like a walking salad.

The months pass and my healing feels like anything but a piece of cake. I am struggling with old demons that have kept my life small and limited for years. Friends consider me brave for not seeing doctors but, in truth, my fear keeps me away: I cannot take the undermining dose of doubt that a trip into the medical world would bring. I decide to learn about macrobiotics so I can understand how it works. I read George Ohsawa's and Michio Kushi's books. I go to the Kushi Institute to study. I sense that my mind is a key element here and I begin to read and study and practice to get it working for me. I make up little ditties about being well and run them through my brain like a broken record to program my subconscious for wellness. I read inspiring stories about others who have healed. My friend Ruska, whose cancer is already gone, suggests we start a support group and so we begin to meet weekly at my house, inviting the local macrobiotic counsellors to be our teachers.

Slowly, sleepily, however, a change begins to take place. I notice differences not just in my body but in the way I think and feel, the way I experience the world. What I have come to understand is this: We are what we eat in ways most of us do not begin to comprehend. By eating whole, balanced, organic foods I am creating a whole, balanced me. Being whole means taking responsibility for our own lives. My hopelessness was stagnation just as much as my cancer was. Clear, holistic thinking is not something we acquire, as if from outside; it is the natural, healthy view that is left when the stagnation goes.

I cannot say that the rough ride became completely smooth after these moments but the journey became progressively easier. Eleven months into my macrobiotic practice I add Chi Gong to my daily regime. Feeling energy course through me — direct experience of the unseen world — makes it real to me and awakens a passion to know more.

In March of 1994, eighteen months after beginning macrobiotics, I decide to have medical testing to see if what Mina has been telling me could be true. A bone scan reveals that the tumor is either in remission or gone and blood work suggests I am cancer free! This might seem like the end of the story but it is not. In macrobiotics we say it takes seven years, give or take, to create a new body. Mind and body are truly one. Spiritual development has been the heart of my healing. I believe that because we are by nature spiritual beings, we are always 'at one' with something. Until my healing from cancer, I was at one with my hopelessness, powerlessness and depression. This path of clearing out my body moved the focus of oneness from myself to what I now call God.

When I was stuck in that old belief system, there was good reason for fear and, in spite of endless attempts, I could not make the fear go away. When I came to understand that I am first and foremost energy/spirit (which happened as good eating began to eliminate the stagnation from my body) and that my body is the result of what is happening on that level of being, then what I believed about healing could change: healing can happen quickly and easily. With these new beliefs, my feelings could change: fear being replaced by love, joy, gratitude, excitement.

People argue over whether the food or the spirit is the primary source of healing. What I know is that while I ate that balanced macrobiotic food, both the cancer and my lifelong depression slipped away. My spirit was able to begin a sleepy awakening that is finally allowing the real me to shine through. My interest in Chi Gong has developed into an intensive study of energy healing and I now have a practice in which I do healing on others, as well as teaching and facilitating self healing. I will forever be indebted to Michio, to Mina, and to all the wonderful macrobiotic teachers who have helped me on my transformational journey.

6. The Case of a Broken Heart

One memorable case was Ivan, who came to America for hope. He was diagnosed with terminal cancer. Neither the surgery, radiation, nor chemotherapy which he received in Yugoslavia helped him. His brother heard about my experience and invited him to try this alternative medicine.

Ivan arrived at my home every morning at 6 a.m. and studied with me until 5 p.m. when he would scurry away like a mouse caught in the light. He was a small man, 60 pounds overweight, spreading at the middle, slow moving and very self-conscious about carrying his colostomy bag. For the most part, he was devoid of smooth creases, having mostly sharp edges. Every dark, luxuriant slicked-down hair was arranged neatly atop his head. His thick, bushy eyebrows dominated his clean shaven face. The expansive condition of his intestines was easily read by his swollen, puffy lips. Obviously, he was a man with a very strong constitution who could potentially live a long life.

Every morning he greeted me with a new story about his last night's dream. Instantly, he became extraordinarily intense. His mouth made a clicking sound, his eyes flashed, his voice deepened. His demeanor changed, while his words cascaded over his lips in impatient swirls. He never ran out of things to say as he allowed himself the sweet pleasure of his newest fantasy.

There he was, in his backyard constructing a three-prong pole securely fastened at the top, with a heavy cast iron pot suspended in the middle above a long burning fire. Cuddled inside the pot was his favorite goulash-paprikash — a spicy pork stew drowned in jalapenos, tomatoes, potatoes, onions, carrots. Or another favorite — a barbecued piglet seasoned with salt and oil. He was rotating his prize and suddenly you would hear him ask in a cool, dispassionate voice, "How long do you cook that rice?"

He had no idea what I was doing in the kitchen, nor did he care about food balance. But in spite of himself, he lost thirty pounds the first month and he started cooking for himself, even balancing correctly. At one point he admitted to actually liking the food and had fewer and fewer "pork" dreams. He was a musician, singing and playing his accordion at weddings. Many times in the middle of our cooking, he would break into song and I would join him. We had an impromptu concert and the meal tasted even better. Believe it or not, people were happier after eating our food, prepared to music.

He never accepted the American way of life. He didn't understand this chaotic lifestyle. He said that Americans make children for "day care" and "baby-sitters." And grandmas and grandpas are in nursing homes. How can a family exist without love? This was his daily complaint to his brother's family. Ivan missed his family. He was desperately homesick, separated from his wife and children. He was here but his heart never was. He didn't understand the time-proven wisdom that macrobiotics is not just about food, even though I was teaching him that every day. He wanted to go back to his country even though it was at war, even if he couldn't find the macrobiotic food he needed.

"I'm not happy here and food cannot make me happy," he protested.

When he started cooking for himself, he was alone in his brother's home all day. His life was empty. Ivan would appear at my home unexpectedly, looking like an unmade bed, saying that he just wanted to talk to someone. Instead of regarding him as an annoyance, our hearts went out to him. His eyes told the truth, dark and knowing, overreached by loneliness. His speech was punctuated by a muffled sadness, unconscious of his grim mood. Sorrow was swelling inside of him, like an ominous black cloud, filling the empty space where happiness once lived. Ivan had no more songs to sing. He was to be pitied.

A year-and-a-half later, on the very day he was scheduled to fly back to Yugoslavia, possessing none of the secrets of immortality, he died but not of cancer, he died of a broken heart.

7. *Guiding Light*
by Ruska Porter

I always believed that I could have a beautiful life but it took six years after being diagnosed with breast cancer to end up living a great life! To say I'm grateful is not enough, particularly when I think of my teachers who taught me how to get where I am now. Mina Dobic is one of them.

Today is November 19th, 1997. On this day six years ago, a doctor told me that I had breast cancer. I felt I was going to faint. My husband turned very pale. "I'm sorry, that you have to go through this once again," I told him. Some time ago, in England, his girl friend had died of breast cancer.

When I look back to that time, I realize how a friendly invisible hand guided me in all my decisions. I chose Dr. Waisman as my oncologist. He was highly recommended and to this day has remained a perfect doctor.

Since I had three lymph nodes involved and unclear margins around the tumor which was Stage II, he recommended removal of the breast, very strong chemotherapy and tamoxifen. It is a drug routinely prescribed for women with breast cancer as a preventative against recurrence.

Very assured that I would find an alternative to my medical cure, I told Dr. Waisman that I would keep my breast, do radiation and weaker chemotherapy. I also told him that I wouldn't take any other drugs after I had completed my treatments. Being as good a doctor as he is, an intuitive person, he knew that he couldn't change my mind and he never tried. He believed that my type of cancer was curable. But he left healing to me.

A while later, when I met with Mina Dobic for a macrobiotic consultation, I found out that we had both worked as journalist/correspondents for the major radio station in Belgrade. Coincidence, one would think: I don't believe so.

During the consultation, she examined every inch of me, which no one had ever done before. I noticed the very special spark in her eyes as she was telling me about the power that grains have for our health, in particular short grain brown rice. A childhood memory came to me: When I was growing up on a little farm in central Bosnia, my grandfather, who was a farmer, used to carry different grains in his pockets as a token of respect for them. When he would sit down with us children (and we were many), he would gently stroke some of the grains in his hands and say, "Look how beautiful and shiny they are." As Mina talked to me about the macrobiotic way of life, she had the same sparks in her eyes as my grandfather did when he talked about his grains. In that split second, I became totally conscious that, from now on, that same light which both of them had in their eyes would be the guiding light in my healing.

That night I went to bed free from worry. I wished that some day by eating grains that light would shine through my eyes as well. The next morning I put several grains of rice in all of my pockets. When I have time, I'll hold them in my hands, so that tradition will go on.

When I was diagnosed with breast cancer, my little country, Bosnia, was going through a war. Since the postal services and telephone lines were shut down, I couldn't write to my mom or telephone her about my illness. And, as sad as this was for me, I knew in my heart that if I told her I was eating grains and vegetables for my healing she wouldn't worry about me. After my grandfather passed away in 1968, my mom was the one who planted grains and vegetables on our land. For many years now, millions of grains had been touched by my mom's hands. What a lovely image I have of my mother in the time of my healing.

In October of 1992, I went to the Kushi Institute for one week of study. Inspired to know more about how to achieve the balance for my new way of life, I went back to Becket for one month every year until I had completed all three levels. Back home in Los Angeles, I continued to study every Thursday night with a wonderful teacher, Cecile Tovah Levin.

For the last five years, every Monday night, Jennifer Greene and I have hosted a Macrobiotic Support Group, one of a kind in Los Angeles. In the first couple of years, Mina gave countless hours of teaching and support to our group.

I go to see Dr. Waisman once a year. Last year I told him that I don't wish to do mammography anymore. He was not surprised and told me so, knowing my new natural style of life.

When I saw him this year in October for blood work only, a week later I received a letter from him.

My Beautiful Life

"Dear Ruska:

I wanted to give you follow-up information on your blood studies which, as usual, were wonderfully normal. Your cholesterol is 162. Congratulations! Your tumor markers, specifically your CA 27-29 and CEA are normal. As you know I continue to urge you to have follow-up mammography but I respect that you are not interested in that."

In so many uncountable ways, life today is beautiful. Even when some real misfortunes happened to me in the last couple of years, I was able to remain calm and focused, feeling that nothing could really push me off center. Perhaps, the beauty of the grains has entered my soul.

Thank you, Mina.

8. A Tennis Champion's Story
by Page Bartelt

April 1998

I thought I ate a very healthy, balanced diet until I was introduced to macrobiotics five months ago. I am training to play professional tennis. I have to be aware of my body, my energy level, how food affects my training and my ability to perform efficiently. My definition of "eating healthy" is: salads, chicken, fruit and low fat dairy products. Despite that healthy menu, I never had enough energy. Often I was sleepy after meals, craving sugar and sweets. Even after sleeping 8 or 10 hours, I woke up feeling tired. Although I waited several hours after eating before practice, an uncomfortable feeling lingered in my body. Food felt like a large lump in the pit of my stomach, still undigested. Usually I attributed this to lack of sleep or overtraining. Or I rationalized: most people feel like this, it's normal.

After switching to eating macrobiotically, immediately I've noticed an enormous increase in energy which is easily sustained throughout the day. I've become more alert. Now I wake up earlier, feeling better with less sleep. My skin is softer and clearer. No more puffy or dark shadows under my eyes. While people around me suffer with a cold or flu, I don't get sick.

Of all these changes, the best is my new-found ability to train harder and excel in my sport. Diet was the only thing I changed. Instantly I was able to practice longer with increased endurance. I don't get nearly as sore after tough matches or long tournaments. My body recovers much faster.

I am sincerely grateful for being introduced to the macrobiotic diet. Each day I feel better. I'm especially thrilled with the improvement in my tennis performance. Most importantly, I believe macrobiotics prevents illness. And I've learned how to promote a sustainable and healthy environment by making better food choices.

9. Ode to Macrobiotics
Anonymous

Mina is very knowledgeable in terms of the relationship between the body and the biochemistry of food. It is most apparent if you've ever spoken with her, or been a patient of Mina's, that she is caring in the deepest and most crucial sense of that word. In the tradition of great physicians, or great artisans of healing, she carries out in no uncertain terms, and executes in no uncertain terms, the ability to do no harm.

When I first came to Mina I was faced with some health challenges. Under the direction of my doctor I had undergone a series of tests, and although the results were not fatal they were challenging nonetheless. I was exhausted as much by the testing as I was by the ailment. Several days later I was introduced to Mina through mutual friends. When Mina arrived at my office she didn't say very much. She looked at me and asked to see my hands. She asked me to take off my shoes so that she could look at my feet. She looked into my eyes and asked me to stick my tongue out further than anyone has ever asked me to stick out my tongue in my life. After that she looked at me, felt my pulse and told me exactly what the 30 days of testing had concluded. I was totally amazed by the insight and accuracy of her diagnosis. In addition, she told me a number of things that I had not been told by my doctor.

She suggested that the body is an extremely wise instrument that can heal itself; it is assisted by the correct and proper diet and the elimination of harmful substances in the body. I followed Mina's advise and found my condition to greatly improve. I was totally astonished by that because I have always been a health food person. At one time I was a vegan vegetarian. I have fasted over the years and I have been on and off several kinds of diets and vegetarian regimes over the years. And although they were gratifying, I have never found a system that was as fully invigorating as macrobiotics.

I see no conflict between my doctor's diagnosis and what Mina has diagnosed through her insight and knowledge

Thank you, Mina

10. Wisdom from Little Beings

Rocky is our neighbor. His family lives across the street from us. One uneventful day in December, he walked slowly up the walkway to my front door, knocked softly and waited for someone to answer. I opened the door and even though he had never before been in my home, he instinctively headed immediately in the direction of my pharmacy — the kitchen.

No one had ever told him I was a macrobiotic counselor. I really don't know what moved him to come to me and I never asked. Nevertheless, his story was not unlike many I had heard. The prognosis was not good. The doctor had opened him up, discovered an abdominal tumor in the pancreas and spleen, pressing against the aorta, causing him to lose feeling in his legs. The doctor sewed him back up and sent him home saying there wasn't much they could do for him. The medication he was taking now only made him worse. He had constant diarrhea, vomited every time he tried to eat, and was losing weight at an alarming rate.

His family had made plans to visit their relatives over the Christmas holiday but Rocky was in no mood to travel. However, at my suggestion, they agreed to let him stay in our home for the next five days while they were away. I assured them he would be feeling better by the time they returned. I prepared medicinal food for him; rice cream and barley cream, seaweed vegetable soup, bean dishes and special condiments with natto (fermented soybeans rich in enzymes and vitamin B-12). Food was served fresh and warm daily. At first he just smelled it but then decided to give this strange-looking concoction a try and quickly gobbled it down. Each meal he seemed to like more than the last, lapping it up, begging for more. I was delighted and encouraged to see such enthusiasm and commitment in someone who had never eaten anything macrobiotic before.

For the next five days he continued to relish every meal, and to our astonishment, was able to keep all the food down. When he first arrived at our door he was dragging himself, his unsteady legs barely supporting his weight, but now it was obvious that his energy level was quickly increasing. He took regular walks and slept peacefully through the night. Rocky by nature is quiet, but his eyes speak volumes. I had only to look into those bright eyes to know how much he genuinely appreciated all that I did for him.

Now almost every day at lunch time Rocky knocks at our door with his palm tree tail! He knows exactly where to find me. When the door opens, in front of us appears the cutest little ashy gray, sooty black, dusty white, curly furred lhasa apso. The mere sight of him tugs at your heart strings. He swaggers into the kitchen. He looks up at me through his long straggly bangs that hide his brown eyes as if to say, "Well, here I am. What's cooking?"

We all take turns cuddling him and he's thrilled. He starts petting each side of his snout with his front paws, melting from all our love and attention. His lunch disappears in one minute and he's asking for more attention. The kids take him outside to play.

"Mom, his legs are straightening up. He's walking much better," Yelena says excitedly.

Srdjan appointed himself in charge of making sure Rocky got his macrobiotic meals delivered. Arame seaweed with corn is one of his favorites, licking the plate clean. For him, this is the best dessert!

Of course, now that Rocky is macrobiotic, he enjoys daily "constitutionals" with regularity. Since he's lost a few pounds, he easily slips through the bars in the fence and runs as fast as he can to our door.

The interesting part of this story is that although we've been neighbors for over a year, Rocky never once came to visit us *until* he got sick! Rocky will never understand what macrobiotics is, yet somehow managed to find me on his own. What he does understand is that this food makes him feel better. And now he refuses to eat what he was eating before. Isn't it interesting that a dog can listen to what his body needs and sets about to find it. Here is a dog teaching us how to find energy in the power of food.

Fortunately, his natural instinct was not destroyed by his synthetic diet. Perhaps this inherent basic instinct possessed by animals guided him. Who knows. Or maybe later there may even be a part for Rocky in Srdjan's movie. After all, he is a hero. He was instrumental in getting his family to consider learning more about the natural way of living and changing their diet to a more healthy one. Could it be said, "Rocky showed them the way?"

11. Motivated by Blood — The Road to Macrobiotics by Phyllis Mueller

My road to macrobiotics was a spotted one (no pun intended). I first heard about it when I hired a friend as an exercise coach. I listened intently as he talked about his experiences and belief in macrobiotics. I tried it but had trouble with the food. Still somehow, I knew I had hit truth. Unfortunately for me, in the early days of my finding macrobiotics, I found only very strict and very untalented cooks. So the food seemed plain and too limiting. But I couldn't sop thinking about it and whenever I did it, I had miraculous beauty and health just permeate this body and the changes were fast, positive and dramatic. But I always fell "off the wagon." I read a lot of books and became convinced it was the way to go but I never actually did it permanently. It was on and off.

After about ten years of more or less thinking about it, I ran into a health problem. I started bleeding pretty heavily, vaginally. I went to a doctor who said I was probably just having a heavy period. But there was so much blood that it would ride up my back to my waist when I was sitting in a chair and I could feel it gushing. That got my attention. I thought I might be bleeding to death right there on the spot. Being leary of "medical" doctors, I went to a doctor who was supposed to be the holistic type. He was recommended to me by a macrobiotic person I trusted, so I did not question the doctor's decision. He took one look at me (during an examination) and said I needed an immediate D & C. Well, before I knew it, I was on that operating table. I got a D & C. Ouch.

When I awoke, the doctor said it went pretty well. There was just one thing… he said he found a growth down there on my left side that he couldn't fully see but he could feel it. It appeared to be the size of a grapefruit and I needed to have another procedure to have it checked out. He said it was probably just a fibroid but it did need to be "checked out right away." Well, after the D & C, I knew I was not going to have another procedure. I was pissed that I'd been bamboozled into a D & C in the first place. What was I thinking? How did this happen when I just wanted some macrobiotic advice?

Anyway, I was worried and frightened. This medical doctor's "grapefruit" comment really got my attention. So this time, I went on macrobiotics pretty strictly. I lost a lot of weight and looked good and never had the problem again. I hung in there for about two years and then slowly fell off the wagon, back to continuing being the mother of all over eaters. Back to sweets, sugar, fat, dairy.

Then came Poland. I was working as a marketing consultant for my own company but on a project for Unisys. The project took us through all of Europe. We were in a different city every day. On this particular day, we were in Poland. Throughout this extended trip, I had not been able to get much to eat except white bread and cheese, with some fruit. This is because I was/am a vegetarian and wherever we went, they served us lots of meat. Well, I won't eat meat, so I'd pick at everything else, mostly the bread and cheese, which I like.

That night, we checked into our hotel and I tried to go to the bathroom. I couldn't. When I looked in the toilet, I was terrified. There was so much blood, I couldn't believe my eyes. I thought I might be having the "heavy period" again. To my horror, I realized I was bleeding from my colon.

The bleeding was so severe that I laid on my stomach on the bed, hoping that gravity would save me. I thought hard about my miserable condition at the time — alone, lonely, bleeding to death in a cold, ugly, dingy hotel in Poland, an almost Communist country at the time, with no one I loved anywhere near me. I knew if Unisys knew what was going on, they'd insist I go to a hospital. That scared me even more. In Poland? As an American, there was no way I was going to a hospital in Poland.

I panicked and placed an SOS call to my husband to call the one macrobiotic counselor I knew. He did and she counselled me through him.

It's funny but without ever speaking to me directly, the instructions I got were to stop eating bread and cheese. How appropriate. Since there wasn't anything else to eat, I just fasted for the next two days. I was frightened and bleeding, so it wasn't hard.

The following morning, I had to give the presentation to the Unisys team, presenting all day, standing up. Unfortunately I was the person making *all* the presentations on this trip. I kept excusing myself and going to the bathroom to see if the blood was running down my legs or showing through my clothes. Fortunately, I had on a dark navy suit and it didn't show a thing. I stuffed extra toilet paper and wash-cloths in my panty hose to soak up the blood. I kept worrying that my client would be horrified if they saw that much blood running down my legs onto their floor. Fortunately, I got through the day without them ever knowing. I told no one.

There's a picture of me at this time, at about 2:45 a.m., taken that night at Poland's Warsaw airport after that all-day meeting. We were leaving Poland that night; as this picture was snapped, I was thinking that this is the picture of a dying woman, who may not even live through this next plane ride. What would people think when they looked at that picture taken minutes before my own death. What was she thinking? Did she have any idea?

So I had a talk with myself. I realized, if I could live through this next day or two by not bleeding to death, I could probably save myself with macrobiotics. But I had to think about the fact that I was still continuing to kill myself with the way I was eating. So I stopped for a minute and had a serious conversation with myself, fully and honestly. I just asked myself, "Do you want to live or do you want to die?" It was clear I was behaving in a manner that was leading to certain death. Why? Why did I want to die so much?

My life was really not that happy. I think I was trying to kill myself in a subconscious sort of way. But then I thought about the impact of my death upon those that do love me. Although I've never really understood why anyone does love me, fortunately, there are those that do. So I thought about those who love me and realized they'd be sad if I died. So I chose, oddly, to live for them. And that worked for me. That gave me enough discipline to clean up my act for another two years or so. I got down to 184 pounds. But slowly, over another few years, I fell completely off the wagon again.

Once fully off the wagon, I quickly put the weight back on and this brings me to the present time. I got back up to 235 pounds. The date is September 14th, 1998. I travel a lot for business. I'd done some heavy travelling for 2–3 weeks, lots of air travel, much more than pilots. Lots of red eyes, my speciality. I got a little cough going. At first, just a throat clearing. Within 24 hours, I had a fever of about 106 and a major case of pneumonia. I could barely stand. Simultaneously, my body decides to pass a few gallstones. Simultaneously, I lose complete control of my bladder and rectum. Simultaneously, I'm weak. Cannot take care of myself. Shaking with cold and fever. Coughing so hard I cannot breathe or sleep. Phlegm in my lungs is dark green and gray with occasional blood. I'm in pain. For those of you who have passed a gallstone or two, you know exactly what I mean.

Now I've been off the macrobiotic wagon for so long, I don't even see anyone macro any more. I mean, I was ashamed to see them since I was obviously back to being a total fool regarding healthy eating. I told my husband that I was pretty sure I was dying right now, at this very moment. I considered going to the hospital but I knew they'd want to remove a minimum of 30% of all my body parts, especially that gall bladder of mine. And I hate doctors. Antibiotics make me even sicker. Again, doctors were just not an option.

So I called in that "macrobiotic bail out counselor" *again*. Her name is Mina Dobic. (Actually she had called me… I think someone close to me put out an SOS call to her on my behalf. I'm not sure about this but the "coincidental timing" is quite miraculous. No one has as yet confessed.)

Wisely I took the call. And can you believe it? With the patience and understanding of Mother Mary, she came to my house and nursed me back to health. My husband stayed home from work two weeks and assisted with this healing process. Needless to say, I was totally unable to care for myself. It took more than a month to fully recover.

This time, though, I had used only macrobiotic food to cure myself. I took no drugs or pain killers of any kind. This time I had not cheated or strayed away from the healing foods. Not one atom of bad food entered this body. In one month, I lost 30 pounds. All of a sudden I was motivated. I'd gotten through some very tough times. I had certainly kicked some bad habits during all that strict healing food. I felt I could take advantage of my position and I did. As an addict I knew I could *not* cheat or I'd be back to peanut butter cups and death. So I decided this time *No cheating.* So far, so good.

Thus, the miraculous discovery I've now made. It's been a great deal easier this time to stick with the program. And it's because I'm *not cheating.*

Now as I write this, the fact that I've had repeated relapses during the two year interval is not lost on me. I know I've got a long road ahead. I know I'm still working to just get to my goal. But I'm confident enough this time. I believe things will be different.

One: I'm writing a book because I feel there is a difference.

Two: I'm not suffering and I had always suffered before.

Three: I love the food now, completely.

Four: I'm winning all the way around with this new approach.

We'll see. We'll just take it one step at a time.

Appendix A
Back to Basics

Scientific Data

January, 1998. Laguna Niguel, California, beautiful USA. My loving family is intact and healthy. I am healed, body, mind and spirit. But I am very concerned because people in America and around the world are sick and getting sicker by the hour. Despite notable strides by the medical research community introducing newly developed therapies and medications, in the United States every 15 seconds someone is diagnosed with heart disease or cancer. For example, at the turn of the century cancer affected one out of twenty-seven people in the United States. By 1950, the rate had leaped to one in eight and by 1985, official estimates were that one out of three people would develop the disease.

If cancer continues increasing at this rate, by the year 2000, every other person could ultimately develop it. By the year 2020, cancer could strike four out of five people and, soon thereafter, virtually everyone!

It was estimated that during the year 1994, more than 520,000 Americans would die of cancer and another 1,130,000 new cases would be detected. Between 1973 and 1988, the incidence of cancer at all sites in the body combined climbed nearly 17 percent (20 percent among men and 13 percent among women). Altogether, according to the American Cancer Society, 83 million Americans now living will eventually get the disease. If this increase continues at the present rate, by the beginning of the twenty-first century 40 to 50 percent of the population will develop cancer during their life and thirty to thirty-five years from now virtually everyone will have the disease at some time before his or her death.

The following startling statistics are evidence of the seriousness of this ever present menace.

CANCER INCIDENCE IN THE UNITED STATES				
	1900	1962	1971	1992
New Cases	25,000	520,000	635,000	1,100,000
Breast	no data	63,000	69,000	175,900
Lung	no data	45,000	80,000	178,000
Colorectal	no data	72,000	75,000	157,500
Prostrate	no data	31,000	35,000	122,000
Uterus	no data	no data	no data	46,000
Persons Affected	1 in 25	1 in 6	1 in 5	1 in 3

An article in the January 9, 1995 issue of *U.S. News & World Report,* (pages 50 and 51), entitled, *A Different Kind of Cancer Risk* says:

"While most drugs are safe and effective when taken as intended, statistics show that up to two million patients are hospitalized each year and as many as 140,000 people die of side effects or reactions related to various prescription drugs. Internal FDA memos obtained by U.S. News reveal enough concern over reported side effects of more than 30 drugs that the agency has placed them on a special list to be watched closely. Used against heart disease, arthritis, infections, asthma, cancer and other common conditions, many of the drugs are taken by millions of people. No one, however, should decide to halt a prescribed medication without talking with a doctor and a pharmacist.

Recent additions to the FDA list include well known and heavily marketed drugs. In November, Paclitaxel, sold by Bristol-Myers Squibb as Taxol for breast and ovarian tumors, was cited because of reports of hypertension. Terazosin, sold by Abbott Laboratories as Hytrin for benign prostate enlargement and hypertension, was added because of reports of priapism — persistent and painful erections that can damage the penis and require emergency treatment. (Abbott would not comment specifically on that report.) The previous month, the arthritis drug oxaprozin (marketed by Searle as Daypro) and the Alzheimer's drug Tacrine (Cognex, from Parke-Davis) came under FDA scrutiny for reports of pancreatitis, or inflammation of the pancreas. A Searle spokesperson says a pancreatitis warning will be added when the Daypro label is reprinted. Parke-Davis says the pancreatitis reports do not appear to be related to Cognex. Aprotinin, a blood coagulant sold by Miles as Trasylol and approved in December 1993 to reduce blood loss during bypass surgery, triggered FDA warning bells last October after at least 16 reported cases of excessive clotting in which 14 of the patients died. In 10 of the 14, death occurred when a blood clot formed in a coronary artery. (Miles says it is "working closely with the FDA" to determine "whether the drug is playing a contributing role.")"

Philosophy

A pamphlet lying on the table attracts my attention. It is entitled *Warning to Humanity*. One thousand, six hundred and seventy top world scientists, including 104 living Nobel Laureates, say: "Human beings and the natural world are on a collision course. Human activities inflict harsh and often irreversible damage on the environment and on critical resources. If not checked... they may so alter the living world that it will be unable to sustain life in the manner that we know. Fundamental changes are urgent if we are to avoid the collision our present course will bring about."

This causes me to reflect. Twenty-six great civilizations are known to have perished but none threatened to take earth-life as we know it with them. The earth and all its people are now confronting the same problem I did as an individual. Cancer is not just one person's problem; it is systemic in our society. "Humanity" is, indeed, "at the Crossroads." Nature or God or whatever or whoever one believes created our Cosmos and all Life is telling us in unmistakable terms: Change your ways of living and thinking and eating — or perish!

The principles of macrobiotics will survive as long as human life survives. Not because it is called "macrobiotics" but because it recognizes and is based on the fact that we are inseparable from nature.

Ohsawa taught that with proper diet we can have a great life, full of adventure, freedom and creativity. He spent the better part of his life spreading macrobiotic philosophy and dietary reform through the world. His students, Michio Kushi, Herman Aihara, Noboru Muramoto and others, modified the diet to accommodate the needs of the Western lifestyle. In this modern time of technological evolution and human "improvement" of what nature has given us, the importance of proper diet for good health has been lost. In some more primitive societies this basic fact was well recognized and used as the basis of medicine.

Macrobiotics' goal is to bring balance to the body and improve the function of our various organs and promote better circulation. It empowers people to make the choices that can prevent degenerative illness and prolong their lives. If disease has already overcome someone, this diet can often halt the process of deterioration and reverse its symptoms. There's a storehouse of books on the subject. There are also countless well-documented personal histories of people who, having been told by their doctors that they were terminally ill, used only macrobiotics to regain their health. One can also find counsellors and teachers of cooking classes, for becoming your own chef is a vital part of healthy living.

In times past, people relied on traditional medicine that was handed down by one generation to the next. Doctors didn't exist. With the natural macrobiotic way, each person comes to realize he is responsible for his own health.

Macrobiotics can be explained as a common sense approach to understanding the relationship between universal law and our environment. That means eating in harmony with the environment to create order and balance in our daily lives. Macrobiotics is not just a Japanese diet, as some people believe. It also represents a philosophy of life. The practice flourished from before the time of Homer to the Renaissance and encompassed all cultures. Essentially it is the diet of common people — laborers, tradesmen, farmers, craftsmen and artists. It is eating whole grains and naturally-grown, non-toxic vegetables, instead of sitting down to a meal of highly processed items out of which most of the living nutrients have been refined.

Food is our most direct connection with nature and sadly we have removed ourselves far from the established order of the universe. The chemicalization and poisoning of food on the land with pesticides; the removal of vital nutrients by refining grains; the overprocessing; the further contamination of foods with additives to prolong shelf life and the often thoughtless way in which we prepare our meals have all taken their toll upon our lives.

Literally, our life is in our own hands. My body will be tomorrow what I chose to eat today. When I finally understood that, I joyfully undertook whatever measures were necessary to save it! Humans are not born cooks.

Why cook food? Aren't raw foods more natural? In the universal sense, fire is every bit as natural as anything else. In the practical sense, it is completely natural for man to use fire in preparing his food, every bit as natural as it is for monkeys to eat their veggies raw.

Man is who he is today because of his use of salt and fire to prepare his food. Through the vehicle of fire and cooking man became man in the true sense of the word. Before that he was no more than a simple beast with a big skull and a very special destiny. Fire is used to change food and tighten up the spirals of fibers in our food and consequently ourselves.

The vegetable kingdom is able to make the great leap across to man. Magnesium must transmute to iron, chlorophyll must become hemoglobin, man must become man. Without cooking this is very difficult to do. There is inefficient transformation without the yin yang energizing force of fire. Eating raw foods tends to cause the charge of the body to become more yin. Consequently the salt expands and discharges the waste, to some degree and in general a cleansing effect is experienced. This can be beneficial at times. In a strong healthy person, it is unnecessary.

By the law of opposites, it is those persons who have overeaten for years that are attracted to fasting. People who have overindulged in sex are drawn to celibacy and folks that are toxic to the extreme insist that we should all be eating raw food, and that fire and salt are evil.

Raw foods weaken blood and discharge cells, which often is a desired effect. They also cause a pleasant cooling effect, best suited to summer. Strong yin food makes the body yin. If people are struggling with any sort of skin problem, avoid raw food altogether. Raw foods are very difficult to digest. Digestive enzymes are not strong enough to break down the fibers of raw food. Undigested food particles sink deep into the corners and crevices of the large intestine, creating dampness and mold (fermentation) and causing the body to become more toxic. Raw food eaters of honey and dairy have parasites and worms which thrive in this creamy, gluey intestinal environment.

So as it turned out, learning to cook was the tool that enabled me to get well. Actually, cooking is the way humans cooperate with nature to form nourishment which creates and sustains life's basic functions. It is a powerful tool which yields either vibrant health, contentment, peace and happiness, or illness, pain, misery and annihilation.

A healthy mind in a healthy body. For thousands of years, wise men and women have taught that this can be achieved by regulation of our diet and daily life and by the quality of our thoughts. It appears that in modern times, many people have forgotten this. However, it is never too late for us to regain this understanding and put it to use to raise our level of health and happiness. The macrobiotic approach to diet and lifestyle is a modern expression of these principles.

The infinite universe is without beginning and without end. It is spaceless and timeless. However, because it is moving in all dimensions at infinite speed it creates phenomena that are infinitesimal and ephemeral. These manifestations have a beginning and an end, a front and a back, measure and duration, and may be viewed as forms appearing and disappearing in an ocean of non-being.

The infinite universe, though itself invisible and beyond the apprehension of the senses, differentiates into two antagonistic but complementary tendencies of centrifugal and centripetal forces, expansion and contraction, time and space, beginning and end, yin and yang.

The terms yin and yang come from the Orient, but a similar understanding is found in some form in most traditional cultures. It is the idea of making harmony between opposites — night and day, light and dark, fast and slow, hot and cold. All objects or activities can be described in terms of yin and yang and are a combination of yin and yang qualities. Thus, no person or object can be completely yang or yin. But one can be more yang or yin than someone or something else. In order to be healthy, we need a balance of both yin and yang traits.

The laws of the universe, in a simplified modern version, can be represented by seven principles of the absolute world and twelve theorems of the relative world, although they are all manifestations of one infinity:

Seven Principles of the Order of the Universe

1. All things are differentiations of One Infinity.

2. Everything changes.

3. All antagonisms are complementary.

4. There is nothing identical.

5. What has a front has a back.

6. The bigger the front, the bigger the back.

7. What has a beginning has an end.

Twelve Theorems of the Unifying Principle

1. One Infinity differentiates itself into yin and yang which are the poles that come into operation when the infinite centrifugal force arrives at the geometric point of bifurcation.

2. Yin and yang result continuously from infinite centrifugal force.

3. Yin is centrifugal. Yang is centripetal. Yin and yang together produce energy and all phenomena.

4. Yin attracts yang. Yang attracts yin.

5. Yin repels yin. Yang repels yang.

6. The force of attraction and repulsion is proportional to the difference of other yin and yang components. Yin and yang combined in varying proportions produce energy and all phenomena.

7. All phenomena are ephemeral, constantly changing their constitution of yin and yang components.

8. Nothing is solely yin or solely yang. Everything involves polarity.

9. There is nothing neuter. Either yin or yang is in excess in every occurrence.

10. Large yin attracts small yin. Large yang attracts small yang.

11. At the extremes, yin produces yang and yang produces yin.

12. All physical forms and objects are yang at the center and yin at the surface.

So what is the meaning of these principles for modern people? How do they apply to our lives?

It is becoming increasingly evident from the deterioration of our planet home that the choices we humans have made are jeopardizing the future of our species and shortening our own lives. Living in the concrete jungles we call cities has taken us far away from the natural world and the order of the universe. In some cases so far away that we hardly know what that natural order is.

We often act without weighing the consequences of our actions. The pesticides we use on food grown for our nourishment poisons us as well as the insects we hope to eradicate. The chemicals which we thoughtlessly or deliberately dispose of in rivers and oceans kills or deforms the fish we used to eat. The acids we release into the atmosphere fall down upon us and our neighbors around the world bringing sickness and devastation with them. It is no accident that degenerative diseases are increasing exponentially.

A basic macrobiotic diet consists of 50% whole grains; 5–10% protein from beans and soybean products; 5–10% sea vegetables; 10% soups, such as miso and 25–30% steamed or fresh organic vegetables.

Short grain brown rice is the preferred grain for daily use; next is whole barley and then millet, rye, buckwheat oats, etc. For the 5% proportion of protein, special beans are recommended: azuki, garbanzo, dark green lentils, black soy beans and soy products such as tempeh, natto and tofu. Soups are usually made with miso and a clear broth with dried shiitake mushrooms and kombu seaweed.

The recommended vegetables are root vegetables such as carrots, burdock and daikon radish; round vegetables, such as cabbage, onion, winter squash and cauliflower and leafy greens, especially kale, broccoli, Chinese cabbage, mustard greens, dandelion, and watercress.

Not recommended are foods containing high levels of potassium and oxalic acid which cause gallstones and kidney stones and draw calcium from the bones. Therefore, it is best to avoid foods of the nightshade family such as tomatoes, potatoes, eggplant, green and red bell peppers.

The occasional supplementary foods include: fish, cooked seasonal fruit, sesame and pumpkin seeds, various natural non-aromatic and non stimulant beverages and various natural processed seasonings and condiments. Some people's condition requires certain natural food home remedies.

To prepare this food properly, you must have good quality cooking utensils. And most important, use gas for cooking. Gas is a natural source and doesn't destroy the molecular structure of the food the way electricity or microwave ovens do. Necessary utensils include stainless steel and seasoned, cast-iron cookware, wooden spoons, etc.

One should have a Dietary Guide with recipes and menus, which gives details on how to carry out this entire program.

My personal experience is a prime example of the effect of modern lifestyle on the human body. I was vaguely aware throughout my adult life that something was missing. I was continuously getting messages: high blood pressure, migraines, PMS, allergies, heartburn, pounding heart, bloating, insomnia, aches and pains all over the body. Unfortunately, like most of my fellow humans, I was too ignorant to decode those signals. We moderns seldom discover the cause of our illness, or any other problem for that matter. Sure, if we have a morning-after hangover and headache, we blame it on too much alcohol. We make that connection. Or if after eating we get nausea and diarrhea, we blame it on the food. We make that connection. But we have no answers for other important questions: Why are we chronically ill? What is the root cause?

The multi-national drug companies are the wealthiest corporations. They hand us potions and pills. Science and the medical profession spend billions of dollars to provide state-of-the-art facilities to treat diseases. But instead, they're faced with new viruses for which they have no cure. On the one hand, we have medicine with all its modern "treatments." On the other hand, out of total deaths, we have ever higher percentages of death from known illnesses such as heart disease, cancer and AIDS. Something is wrong.

We have no answer because we don't make the right connection. If we can make the connection between too much alcohol and a hangover or food poisoning and diarrhea, what prevents us from making the larger connection? The connection is not made because "civilized" people have forgotten we are inseparable from nature. We are nature. But the connection wasn't made with the many years of eating a diet consisting of beef, pork, chicken, cheese, ice cream, milk and all the chemicals in those foods; too much salt, oil, candies, cakes, fruit, juices, sugar, alcohol and drugs. Not only has this been our menu of choice but our parents and their parents made the very same food selections! They were as sick as we are. Maybe they died because they did not know how to treat themselves.

Regularly-consumed, these foods create cysts and tumors in the reproductive organs: dairy products like milk, cheese, ice cream; chocolate, soft drinks, sugar and other sweeteners; fruit and fruit juices; nut butters; greasy and oily foods; refined flour products such as pastries, croissants, doughnuts and sweet rolls; hamburgers and other animal foods. That's not even saying anything about the chemical additives added to our so-called "food". Oh, God, I'll starve to death!

How do you eliminate serious reproductive illnesses? Just stop whatever you've been doing! Center your diet on whole grains, beans, vegetables, sea vegetables and small amounts of fruit and seeds.

Recently, some cancer specialists have linked the spread of genital herpes virus to cervical cancer. They consider it precancerous. It is not, they say, caused by any outside virus. The true cause is food high in fat and sugar. In contrast, eating whole foods creates balanced nutrition which produces good quality blood. This enables the immune system to effectively eliminate bacteria and other microorganisms.

So then, if we can make the connection that by eating certain foods we make ourselves sick, can we make the more important connection, namely that if we eat certain other foods, nature will heal us? If our body needs vitamins, minerals and supplements, then why not select these nutrients from better quality foods from natural sources that strengthen our immune system? That's the right connection. That's the connection we should be making. To that we should be paying full attention. That's what we should be studying. That's the answer!

We go to doctors hoping they'll find the cause of our illness and know how to treat it. It may take us awhile, but if we're among the few fortunate ones, we finally realize they don't have the answer either. Sad to say, more and more people are dying from the same diseases.

Of course, I didn't know it then, but I know it now. Everything we put in our mouth feeds our blood. Our bloodstream carries the blood to every organ of the body. One of the first things you learn in Chinese medicine is that the utmost important bodily function is good blood circulation. The Chinese call it Ki. In healthy people, blood travels throughout the body ten miles every hour. If blood travels throughout the body only five miles every hour, that means the person is very weak. Blood transports iron to nourish us. If the supply of iron is depleted or insufficient, the result is weakness, low energy level, anemia.

The standard macrobiotic diet is based not only on nutritional balance but also on a deep understanding of biological and spiritual evolution; environmental atmospheric conditions; the relationship of the earth to the sun and other essential bodies; and other factors.

Today macrobiotics is a harmonious blend of East and West. We can adopt its principles in our everyday life by selecting food from organic produce and applying various cooking styles according to our constantly changing individual needs. Two books that give an excellent overview of the subject are: *The Macrobiotic Way* by Michio Kushi and *The Complete Guide to Macrobiotic Cooking* by Aveline Kushi.

The standard macrobiotic diet, like a custom-made suit, can be specifically designed to meet each person's individual needs with respect to age, sex, activity, cultural background, constitution and condition. It varies according to the climate, season, temperature, atmosphere, and where we live. For instance, in California which has a two-season climate, the dietary approach will be different than that for the East Coast with a four-season climate.

This is why I have become a macrobiotic counselor and cook. I want to share my knowledge in the hopes of sparing others the pain of learning the hard way as I had to do.

The order of the universe is the order of balance and harmony, or in other words, love. Vibrant health is realized by bringing our view of life into direct alignment with natural order. Once we no longer regard sickness as an enemy but rather as an opportunity to discover a deeper meaning in health, we can more fully love ourselves and others. Discovering who we are and loving ourselves, heartfelt appreciation and genuine acceptance, are the enduring foundation for lasting health. Thus, we can then be at peace with ourselves and the world.

Appendix B

Menu Used by Mina Dobic to Heal Her Cancer

Monday Menu

Breakfast: 8:00 a.m.

Miso Soup: onion, carrots, cabbage, mochi, wakame seaweed, 1 sheet of nori

Grain: short grain brown rice, with kombu, 2 slices home-made pickles

Steamed Greens: carrots w/tops

At 11:30 a.m. Sweet Vegetable Drink made of $1/2$C each: onion, carrots, green cabbage, squash

Lunch: 12:30 p.m.

Grain: short grain rice and whole barley, with kombu, 2 slices of pickle

Protein Dish: winter squash, azuki beans with kombu

Pressed Salad: cabbage with red radishes, sea salt, brown rice vinegar

Steamed Greens: collards

At 4 p.m. Azuki Bean Tea

Dinner: 5:30 p.m.

Clear Broth Soup : with broccoli

Grain: 70% short grain brown rice, 20% sweet rice, 10% dried chestnuts, 2 slices of pickle

Arame seaweed: with onion, carrots

Steamed Greens: kale

Drink of Bancha Twig tea, only if thirsty

TUESDAY MENU

Breakfast: 8:00 a.m.

Miso Soup:	daikon with tops, wakame seaweed, shiitake mushroom, 1 sheet of Nori
Soft Grain:	millet with winter squash, 2 slices of pickle
Steamed Greens:	green cabbage with parsley
Noon:	1 C Sweet Vegetable Drink

Lunch: 12:30 p.m.

Grain:	short grain brown rice with rye, 2 slices of pickle
Protein Dish:	dark green lentil stew
Boiled Salad:	cabbage, red radishes, broccoli, with sesame dressing
At 4 p.m.	Azuki Bean Tea

Dinner: 5:30 p.m.

Clear Broth Soup:	leeks, carrots, savoy cabbage
Grain:	short grain brown rice with azuki beans, 2 slices of pickle
Nishime:	daikon, carrots, dry lotus root, cabbage, kombu
Steamed Greens:	daikon tops
At 7:30 p.m.	Daikon-Carrot Drink

WEDNESDAY MENU

Breakfast: 8:00 a.m.

Miso Soup:	leeks, brussels sprouts, carrots, 1 sheet of Nori
Soft Grain:	short grain brown rice with kombu, 2 slices of pickle
Steamed Greens:	cabbage with carrot tops
Medicinal Drink:	Ume-Sho-Kuzu
Noon:	Sweet Vegetable Drink

Lunch: 12:30 p.m.

Grain:	short grain brown rice with winter wheat, 2 slices of pickles
Protein Dish:	chickpea stew: onion, carrots, squash
Boiled Salad:	red radishes with tops, Chinese cabbage, kale
At 4 p.m.	Black Soy Bean Juice

Dinner: 5:30 p.m.

Nabe Dish:	kombu, shiitake mushrooms, daikon with tops, parsnips, leeks, lotus root, carrots

2 slices of pickles
Daikon-Carrot Drink

THURSDAY MENU

Breakfast: 8:00 a.m.
Miso Soup: onion, squash, mochi, parsley, 1 sheet of Nori
Soft Grain: millet with pumpkin seeds, 2 slices of pickles
Steamed Greens: collards, Chinese cabbage
Medicinal Drink: Ume-Sho-Kuzu
At noon: Sweet Vegetable Drink

Lunch: 12:30 p.m.
Grain: 80% short grain brown rice, 20% hato mugi, kombu, 2 slices of pickles
Protein Dish: black soybean stew
Pressed Salad: cabbage, celery, red radishes
At 4 p.m.   Black Soybeans: onion, rutabaga, parsley

Dinner: 5:30 p.m.
Squash Soup: winter squash, onion, parsley
Grain: short grain brown rice, sweet rice, kombu, 2 slices of pickles
Hiziki: with onion, dried daikon, carrots
Steamed Greens: collards
Daikon-Carrot Drink

FRIDAY MENU

Breakfast: 8:00 a.m.
Miso Soup: daikon, celery, wakame, shiitake mushroom, 1 sheet of Nori
Soft Grain: soak whole oats overnight, 2 slices of pickle
Steamed Greens: green cabbage with carrot tops
Medicinal Drink: Ume-Sho-Kuzu
At noon: Sweet Vegetable Drink, 1 C

Lunch: 12:30 p.m.
Grain: millet mashed like potato with cauliflower, 2 slices of pickle
Protein Dish: tempeh, dried daikon, onion, carrots
Pressed Salad: cabbage, red radishes with tops, umeboshi vinegar
Steamed Greens: kale
At 2 p.m. $1/2$C Shiitake Tea

Dinner: 5:30 p.m.
Barley Soup: onion, parsnips, cabbage, shiitake mushroom, kombu
Udon noodles
2 slices of pickles
Quick Water Saute: leeks, Chinese cabbage, carrots, snow peas
Steamed Greens: collards
At 4 p.m.   Azuki Bean Tea

SATURDAY MENU

Brunch: 10:30 a.m.

Miso Soup:	onion, cabbage cauliflower, wakame seaweed, mochi, 1 sheet of Nori
Grain:	short grain brown rice with umeboshi plum, 2 slices of pickles
Hiziki:	with winter squash, kombu
Boiled Salad:	carrots, broccoli, white part of leeks, with pumpkin seed dressing
Sweet Vegetable Drink	1 C
At 3 p.m.	$1/_2$C Shiitake Tea

Dinner: 5:00 p.m.

Nabe Dish:	collard, Chinese cabbage, cauliflower, shiitake mushrooms, kombu, tofu
Udon noodles	
2 slices of pickle	
Kinpira:	onion, burdock, carrots, lotus root
At 6:30 p.m.	Daikon-Carrot Drink

SUNDAY MENU

Brunch: 10:30 p.m.

Miso Soup:	leeks, turnip, cabbage, wakame, 1 sheet of Nori
Grain:	short grain brown rice, sweet rice, chestnuts, roasted black soybeans, 2 slices of pickle
Pressed Salad:	Chinese cabbage, carrots, kale, parsley with umeboshi dressing
Sweet Vegetable Drink:	1C
If hungry:	eat sushi for a snack

Dinner: 5:00 p.m.

Nabe Dish:	daikon, carrots, Chinese cabbage, kombu, shiitake mushroom, collards
Steamed winter squash:	with mochi
2 slices of pickles	
$1/_2$C Shiitake Tea	

HOME REMEDIES — INTERNAL TREATMENTS

Ume Sho Kuzu

1. Dilute one heaping teaspoon of kuzu with a couple teaspoons of water.
2. Add diluted kuzu to 1 cup of water.
3. Add the meat of $1/3$ umeboshi plum to the water and kuzu.
4. While bringing to a boil, stir constantly to avoid lumping. Reduce flame and simmer until it is translucent.
5. Add $1/3$ tsp. of shoyu, (soy sauce, alcohol free) and stir. Simmer 30 seconds longer and drink hot.

Carrot/Daikon Drink

1. Grate $1/2$ cup of carrots, plus $1/2$ cup of daikon or black radish.
2. Add 2 cups of water and simmer 4 minutes. Add 4 drops of shoyu while simmering.

Sweet Vegetable Drink

1. Use $1/2$ cup each of four sweet vegetables, finely chopped. (Onions, carrots, cabbage and sweet winter squash; in season, add corn.)
2. Boil four times the amount of water, add chopped vegetables and allow to boil, uncovered for 2–3 minutes. Reduce flame to low, cover and let simmer for 20–30 minutes.
3. Strain the vegetables from the broth. (You may occasionally use them later in soups and stews.)
4. Drink the broth, either hot or at room temperature.

No seasoning is used in this recipe. Sweet vegetable broth may be kept in the refrigerator for up to two days but should be warmed again or allowed to return to room temperature before drinking.

Azuki Bean Tea

Good for regulation of kidney and urinary functions. Helpful for smooth bowel movement.
1. Place one cup of beans in a pot with 2" kombu (soaked and finely chopped).
2. Add four cups of water and bring to a boil
3. Lower the flame, cover and simmer for approximately 30 minutes.
4. Strain out the beans and drink the liquid while hot.
5. You may continue cooking the beans longer with additional water until soft and edible or combine them with other recipes.

Black Soy Bean Tea

1 cup black soy beans   2" burdock   2" sliced lotus root
1 lg. shiitake mushroom   1/3 cup dried daikon 1 umeboshi plum
6 cups water

Simmer 45 minutes with cover ajar. Strain juice. Bring back to boil. Add umeboshi plum, chopped. Simmer 5 min.

Shiitake Mushroom Tea

Traditionally known to reduce fever, help dissolve animal quality fat and help relax a contracted or tense condition.

1. Soak one shiitake mushroom in one cup of water for 20 to 30 minutes.
2. When shiitake mushroom is soft, chop finely.
3. Bring to boil.
4. Reduce flame to gentle simmer for 10 to 15 minutes.
5. Add a pinch of sea salt or few drops of shoyu/soy sauce toward the end.
6. Drink while hot.

Note: For children one year old or younger do no add any seasoning to the tea.

Daikon Drink No. 1

Will help to lower fevers by inducing sweat. Good also to give relief from poisoning caused by meat, fish or shell fish.

1. Grate about 3 T of fresh daikon.
2. Mix daikon with 1/4 tsp. grated ginger and 1/2 tsp. sea salt or 1T shoyu/soy sauce.
3. Pour 2 to 3 cups of hot bancha twig stem tea over the mixed ingredients.
4. Drink as much of the tea as possible while hot.
5. After drinking this tea, go to bed and wrap yourself in a blanket to induce perspiration.

Notes:
*   This tea is very strong — do not take more than twice a day for one or two days.
*   For children, limit the quantity to one half cup per day.
*   To reduce fever in babies and young children, it is better to give apple juice, grated apple or a kuzu drink with rice syrup. Dissolve one tsp. of kuzu in cold water. Add one tsp. of rice syrup. Bring to a gentle boil over a medium flame while stirring and turn off the flame as soon as the drink has thickened and become translucent.

Bancha Tea

1. Place $^1/_2$ to 2 T of roasted twigs in $1^1/_2$ quarts of spring water. Bring to boil. Keep unused twigs in air tight jar until needed.
2. When the water boils, reduce flame to low and simmer for several minutes. For a light tea, simmer 2 to 3 minutes. For a darker, stronger tea simmer 10 to 15 minutes.
3. To serve, place a small bamboo or metal tea strainer in each cup and pour out the tea. Twigs in the strainer may be returned to the tea pot and reused several times.
4. Bancha tea may be served hot year-round as well as cool in summer. It is usually drunk plain. Although for medicinal purposes, a drop of tamari or shoyu/soy sauce may be mixed in.

HOME REMEDIES — EXTERNAL

Daikon Hip Bath

Warms the body; treats womens' reproductive organs, treats skin problems, aids in extracting body odors due to consumption of animal foods; draws out excess fat and oil from the body.

Dry fresh daikon leaves in a shady place until they are brown and brittle. If daikon leaves are not available, however, use turnip leaves or a handful of arame seaweed.

1. Place about 4 to 5 bunches of dried leaves in a large pot.
2. Add about 4 to 5 quarts of water and bring to a boil.
3. Reduce to a medium flame and boil the leaves until the water is brown.
4. Add a handful of sea salt and stir well to dissolve.
5. Pour the hot liquid into a small tub. Add water until the bath level is waist high when sitting in the tub.
6. Keep the temperature as hot as possible and keep the body covered with a large towel.
7. Take the bath for 15 to 20 minutes, preferably just before bedtime but at least one hour after eating.

Note: Keep the hip area warm after coming out of the bath.

Tofu–Chlorophyl Plaster

Helps concussions, fevers, burns; in many cases it is much more effective than ice.

1. Squeeze out liquid from tofu, mash the tofu and mix about 10 to 20% unbleached white flour and 5% grated ginger.
2. Chop several green leafy vegetable leaves (collards, kale, etc.) very finely.
3. Place in a suribachi and grind.
4. Mix all ingredients together.
5. Apply the plaster directly to the skin about $1/2$ inch thick, place a towel over it and tie it in place so it doesn't move.
6. Change the plaster every 2 to 3 hours or when it becomes hot.

LIFESTYLE SUGGESTIONS AND HOME CARE

1. Body Scrub — with a towel dipped in hot water (squeezed out) once a day in the morning.

2. Body Scrub — with a towel dipped in hot ginger water (squeezed out) once a day in the evening before bed. Follow with a 17 second shower.

   (A body scrub should be separate from your bath or shower (either before or after). Baths and showers should be kept short for optimum health.)

3. Walking outside in the fresh air for one half hour or longer is very beneficial for improving health.

4. Exercise or sports, in moderation, are also beneficial.

5. Please wear only 100% cotton clothing.

6. Use 100% cotton for all bedsheets and pillow cases.

7. Keep several green plants in your home to freshen and improve the condition of the indoor air.

For best health, it is advisable to avoid or minimize the following:

1. Watching TV for long periods. (Limit to about one half-hour each day).

2. Using computers for long periods.

3. Using fluorescent lights in your home or workplace.

4. Being exposed to a chemicalized environment.

5. Using artificially chemicalized cosmetics, soaps, toothpaste, etc. Toiletries made from more natural ingredients are available from your natural food store.

SPECIAL COOKING SUGGESTIONS

For optimum health, we recommend the following:

1. Use pots and pans of stainless steel, ceramics and/or cast iron, rather than aluminum cookware.

2. Cook with gas or wood rather than electricity. Especially avoid microwave cooking.

3. Minimize baking foods in the oven.

4. Eat regularly in a relaxed manner, two or three meals a day as desired.

5. Late night eating or snacking is not recommended. It is best not to eat for three hours before sleeping.

6. Each meal should be centered around grains, 50% or more.

7. Variety in the selection and methods of preparation of various kinds of dishes is very important. Please keep in mind that a strict diet does not mean a narrow diet.

Maintain a happy, relaxed and regular lifestyle. And most of all, sing a happy song!

Glossary

Agar Agar – A gelatin processed from a sea vegetable used in making kanten and vegetable aspics.

Amasake – A sweet, creamy beverage or sweetener made from fermented sweet rice.

Arame – A thin, wiry black sea vegetable.

Azuki Bean – A small, dark red bean originally from Japan but now grown in the West.

Bancha Tea – The twigs, stems and leaves from mature Japanese tea bushes, also known as kukicha.

Barley – A whole cereal grain; the traditional staple of the Middle East and Southern Europe.

Boiled Salad – A salad whose ingredients are lightly boiled or dipped (blanched) in hot water before serving.

Bok Choy – A leafy green and white vegetable popular in Chinese cooking.

Bonito Flakes – Flakes shaved from dried bonito fish. Used in soup stocks or as a garnish.

Brown Rice – Whole unpolished rice. Come in three main varieties: short, medium and long grain. Brown rice contains an ideal balance of nutrients and.is the principal staple in macrobiotic cooking.

Burdock – A hardy wild plant that grows throughout the United States and abroad. The long, dark root is valued in cooking for its strengthening qualities.

Daikon – A long white radish that is used in vegetable cooking, condiments and pickling.

Flame Deflector – A round metal disc that is placed under a pot or pressure cooker to distribute heat evenly and prevent burning.

Ginger – A spicy, pungent golden colored root used in cooking and for medicinal purposes.

Gomashio – Sesame seed salt made from dry roasting and grinding sea salt and sesame seeds and crushing in a mortar.

Hato Mugi or Pearl Barley – This is not the so called "pearled" barley, a kind of refined barley. It is not really a barley at all. It is a pearl shaped seed of wild grass, also known as "Job's tears".

Hiziki – A dark brown sea vegetable that turns black when dried.

Hokkaido Pumpkin – A round dark green or orange squash that is very sweet and harvested in the fall. Native to New England, it was introduced to Japan and named after the island of Hokkaido.

Kanten – A jelled fruit dessert made from agar agar.

Kinpira – A style of cooking root vegetables first by sautéing, then adding a little water, and seasoning with tamari/soy sauce at the end of cooking.

Kombu – A wide, thick, dark green sea vegetable.

Kuzu – A white starch made from the root of a prolific vine. Used as a thickener for soups, stews, desserts. Also known as kudzu.

Lotus Root – Root of the water lily. Brown-skinned with a hollow, chambered off-white inside. Lotus root is used in many dishes and for medicinal preparations.

Millet – A small yellow grain that can be prepared whole, added to soups, salads and vegetable dishes, or baked. A staple in China and Africa.

Mirin – A sweet cooking wine made from sweet rice.

Miso – A fermented pate made from soybeans, sea salt and usually rice or barley. Used in soup, stews and as seasoning.

Mochi – A cake made from cooked, pounded sweet rice.

Nabe – A traditional Japanese one-dish meal, prepared and served in colorful casserole dishes and accompanied with a dipping sauce or broth made of tamari/soy sauce or miso and various garnishes.

Natto – Soybeans that have been cooked and mixed with beneficial enzymes and fermented for 24 hours. A sticky dish with long strands and a strong odor. Good for improving digestion.

Nishime – Long, slow style of boiling in which vegetables or other ingredients cook primarily in their own juices. Gives strong, peaceful energy.

Nori – Thin sheets of dried sea vegetable. Black or dark purple, they turn green when roasted over a flame. Used as a garnish, to wrap rice balls, in making sushi, or cooked with tamari/soy sauce as a condiment.

Pressed Salad – Salad prepared by pressing sliced vegetables and sea salt in a small pickle press or with an improvised weight.

Pressure cooker – An airtight metal pot that cooks food quickly by steaming under pressure at a high temperature. Used primarily in macrobiotic cooking for whole grains and occasionally for beans and vegetables.

Rice Syrup – A natural sweetener made from malted brown rice.

Sea Salt – Unrefined salt obtained from the ocean.

Seitan – A whole wheat product cooked in shoyu, kombu and water. Used for stews, croquettes, etc. Also known as wheat gluten or wheat meat.

Shiitake – A mushroom native to Japan but now cultivated in the United States as well. Used widely, dried or fresh, in cooking, for soups and stews and in medicinal preparations.

Shoyu – Naturally made soy sauce.

Soba – Noodles made from buckwheat flour or buckwheat combined with whole wheat.

Suribachi – A serrated, glazed clay bowl or mortar. Used with a pestle, called a surikogi, for grinding and pureeing food.

Tamari – "Genuine" or "real tamari" is a soy sauce like seasoning that is a by-product of the miso making process. It is stronger than regular shoyu or natural soy sauce, which is sometimes confusingly labelled "tamari soy sauce."

Tempeh – A high protein soy product made from split soybeans, water and a special bacteria. Used in soups, stews, sandwiches and many other dishes.

Tekka – Condiment made from matcho miso, sesame oil, burdock, lotus root, carrot and ginger root. It cooks down to a black powder when sautéed on a low heat for several hours.

Tofu – Soybean curd made from soybeans and nigari (crystallized residue from sea salt). High in protein and usually prepared in the form of cakes that may be sliced and cooked in soups, vegetable dishes, salads, sauces, dressings and other styles.

Udon – Japanese style whole wheat noodles.

Umeboshi – A salted pickled plum usually aged for several years. Used as a seasoning, in sauces, and as a condiment.

Umeboshi Vinegar – Also known as ume-su. The liquid that umeboshi plums are aged in. Used for sauces, dressings, seasoning and making pickles.

Wakame – A long, thin green sea vegetable used in making miso soup, salads and vegetable dishes.

Bibliography

Andric, Ivo. *Ex Ponto*. Sarajevo, 1981.

Aihara, Cornellia and Herman with Carl Ferre. *Natural Healing from Head to Toe*. Avery Publishing Group, Inc., Garden City Park, New York, 1994.

Kohler, Jean Charles and Mary Alice. *Healing Miracles from Macrobiotics: A Diet for all Diseases*. Parker Publishing Co., Inc., West Nyack, N.Y., 1979.

Kushi, Michio. *Visions of a New World: The Era of Humanity*. Published by the East West Journal, Inc., Brookline, Massachusetts, 1980.

Kushi, Michio. *How to See Your Health: Book of Oriental Diagnosis*. Japan Publications, Inc., Tokyo - New York, 1980.

Kushi, Michio with Olivia Oredson. *Macrobiotic Palm Healing*. Japan Publications, Inc., Tokyo and New York, 1988.

Kushi, Michio with Edward Esko. *Spiritual Journey*. One Peaceful World Press, Becket, Massachusetts, 1994.

Kushi, Michio with Edward Esko. *The Macrobiotic Approach to Cancer*. Avery Publishing Group, Inc., Garden City Park, New York, 1991.

Kushi, Michio. Edited by Marc Van Cauwenberghe, M.D. *Macrobiotic Home Remedies*. Japan Publications, Inc., Tokyo and New York, 1985.

Kushi, Michio. Edited by Alex Jack. *Standard Macrobiotic Diet*. One Peaceful World Press, Becket, Massachusetts, 1996.

Kushi, Michio with Alex Jack. *One Peaceful World*. St. Martin's Press, New York, 1987.

Kushi, Michio with Alex Jack. *Diet for a Strong Heart*. St. Martin's Press, New York, 1985.

Kushi, Michio with Alex Jack. *The Cancer Prevention Diet*. Revised and Updated. St. Martin's Griffin, New York, 1994.

Kushi, Michio and Aveline. Compiled with the help of Edward Esko, Murray Snyder, Bill Spear and Bill Tara. *Macrobiotic Dietary Recommendations*. Published by Macrobiotic Association of Connecticut, 1987.

Kushi, Michio. *Your Face Never Lies*. Avery Publishing Group, Inc., Wayne, New Jersey, 1983.

Kushi, Michio and Aveline. *Macrobiotic Diet*. Japan Publications, Inc., Tokyo and New York, 1985.

Kushi, Aveline with Alex Jack. *Macrobiotic Cooking: For Health, Harmony and Peace.* Warner Books, New York, 1985.

Mann, Thomas. *The Magic Mountain. First Vintage International Edition.* Translated from German by John E. Woods. Alfred A. Knopf, Inc., New York, 1995.

Ohsawa, George. *An Invitation to Health & Happiness.* George Ohsawa Macrobiotic Foundation, Oroville, California, 1971.

Ohsawa, George. *The Book of Judgment: The Philosophy of Oriental Medicine, Volume 2.* George Ohsawa Macrobiotic Foundation, Oroville, California, 1984.

Ohsawa, George. *Macrobiotics: The Way of Healing.* (Formerly titled *Cancer and the Philosophy of the Far East,* 1971). George Ohsawa Macrobiotic Foundation, Oroville, California, 1984.

Directories

Macrobiotic Resource Guide
One Peaceful World
Box 10
Becket, MA 01223
Phone: (413) 623-2322
Fax: (413) 623-6042

The International Macrobiotic Directory
by Robert Mattson
1050 40th Street
Oakland, CA 94608
Phone: (510) 601-1763

Acknowledgments

There is no way to thank all the people whose lives have touched mine and thereby contributed to the essence of this book. But if I were to single out a few it would be Michio and Aveline Kushi. Michio was destined to be a philosopher, a teacher and a healer. Aveline has so generously shared her culinary secrets with the world. She is a powerful, humble and a genuine human being who has devoted herself to encouraging the human potential. A woman from whom I have learned the Gospel of life. I am extremely honored to know them and have them as my teachers.

Alex Jack is a dear friend, brilliant writer and prolific author whose experience, insight and encouragement helped me set the direction for this manuscript. I am grateful for his writing skill which influenced my writing style and shaped me into an even better writer.

It constantly amazes me how the universe sends into our lives exactly the right people at exactly the right time to help us fulfil our dreams. This happened to me three years ago when a petite dynamo named Tiffany Joy Gates appeared in one of my classes at the San Diego School of Healing Arts. Instinctively we sensed that one day we would do something "big" together, and we did! This book couldn't have been written without her.

TJ, as she is fondly known, became my student and assistant. As I recalled the joys and sorrows of my life, TJ helped substitute the right English words for my Yugoslav expressions. She also gifted me with poetic phrases and wisdom from her own experience. Our work together was pure joy.

Al Lewis and Suzanne Phillips joined us as editors. Suzanne is an accomplished writer and structured the book to focus its impact. A. J. Lewis, Ph.D., psychotherapist and leader in the human potential movement, dreams of a planet which "yet shall bloom with gardens nurtured by the hand of man...." His ability to identify the thrust of a paragraph and select the most poignant words was an incredible asset.

Phyllis Mueller and Glenn Warren gave me a jump start with this book. I thank you for your never-ending support and friendship.

Branca Kojic, my closest friend never said "no" to any of my requests to assist in translating my notes into poetic English.

Mira Drinchich, a beautiful, loving and caring friend, helped me translate some linguistically difficult portions of my manuscript.

Milena Markovich, my special friend, who became part of our family. Many thanks for preparing all those delicious macro meals which allowed me time to work on this book.

Thanks to my computer guides Srdjan, Bruce Cooper and Glenn Warren, who more than once bailed me out of trouble.

A book will never be printed without a publisher. My heartfelt thanks to Diane Mills who introduced me to Findhorn Press. I am grateful to their editor, Tony Mitton, and all their staff who helped this volume see the light of day.

Gratitude to my loving husband and children is expressed throughout the book.

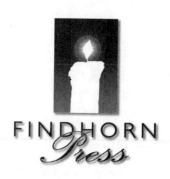

FINDHORN Press

Findhorn Press is the publishing business of the Findhorn Community which has grown around the Findhorn Foundation in northern Scotland.

For further information about the Findhorn Foundation and the Findhorn Community, please contact:

Findhorn Foundation
The Visitors Centre
The Park, Findhorn IV36 3TY, Scotland, UK
tel 01309 690311• fax 01309 691301
email reception@findhorn.org
www.findhorn.org

For a complete Findhorn Press catalogue, please contact:

Findhorn Press

The Park, Findhorn,
Forres IV36 3TY
Scotland, UK
Tel 01309 690582
freephone 0800-389 9395
Fax 01309 690036

P. O. Box 13939
Tallahassee
Florida 32317-3939, USA
Tel (850) 893 2920
toll-free 1-877-390-4425
Fax (850) 893 3442

e-mail info@findhornpress.com
findhornpress.com

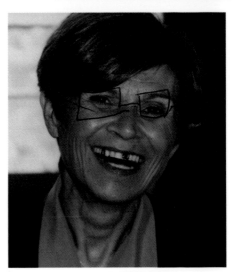

In 1987 Mina was diagnosed with stage IV ovarian cancer with metastases to the liver and lymph system: she was given two months to live. She declined the doctors recommendation for chemotherapy and radiation, and decided to adopt the macrobiotic way of life and healing diet. Six and a half months later she was cancer free.

Milenka "Mina" Dobic, Ph.D. was born in former Yugoslavia in October 15, 1942. She became a professor of Linguistics and World Literature, and later Director of Art and Education for *Radio Indjije*, *Radio Belgrade*, and *Radio Navi Sad*. She was honored with the highest award given in journalism, *The Truth* (equivalent of the Pulitzer Prize).

Mina and her family arrived in the USA in 1987 where she became a teacher and counselor at the Kushi Institute. She later organized the first macrobiotic support group for cancer survivors in Hollywood and has been leading seminars in Nutritional Sciences, Food Sciences and Human Nutrition. In 1998 she was appointed by the Kushi Institute to serve as its Representative at The First Annual Whole World Health Forum. She is currently lecturing nationally and conducting monthly Macrobiotic Cooking Classes for Executive Chefs and others at The Ritz-Carlton Hotel in Dana Point, California.

Health • Nutrition • Biography

Mina Dobic is an intuitive woman committed to the liberation of humanity and One Peaceful World. Growing from patient to healer and motivated by a sincere desire to fulfill her goal, she taught thousands how to transform their sicknesses and misery into health, happiness and peace.

Michio Kushi acknowledged leader of the International Macrobiotic Community and Natural Foods Movement

Mina's story of her life is moving as well as amazing. Her journey from Yugoslavia to California and how she overcame her own cancer, has inspired others who are sick to seek her help. Her healing advice has seen me through many of my illnesses with her love, compassion and insights.

Dr. Benjamin Spock, Pediatrician and Author

Five years ago, in good health I became macrobiotic. Four years ago, I met Mina and through her precise and caring guidance I began to finally really live, not only exist. God Bless you, Mina.

Monty Montgomery, Hollywood Producer, Writer, Director

I am overwhelmed by the beauty, insight, and courage of this book. Mina is a special kind of healer. This book will give you a wonderful tool for maintaining your health. It will also give you a refreshing and insightful way of looking at any health challenge.

Bill Duke, Hollywood Director, Actor, Author

Mina Dobic is widely considered L. A.'s most expert macrobiotic health consultant.

Vogue Magazine, May 1997

Mina truly is in the business of saving lives through changes in lifestyles and healthy eating. The results are dramatic and indisputable.

Ashley Goodwin, Manager of Special Events, The Ritz-Carlton, Laguna Niguel

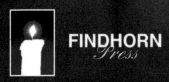

FINDHORN
Press

$15.95
£9.95

ISBN 1-899171-13-4

9 781899 171132